Healing Crisis and Trauma With Mind, Body, and Spirit

Barbara Rubin Wainrib, EdD

BAKER COLLEGE OF
CLINTON TWP. LIBRARY

D1310695

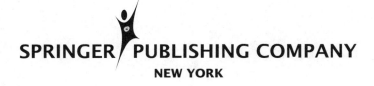

SPRINGER PUBLISHING COMPANY
NEW YORK

Copyright © 2006 by Springer Publishing Company, Inc.

All rights reserved.

No part of this publication may be reproduced, stored in a retrieval system, or transmitted in any form or by any means, electronic, mechanical, photo-copying, recording, or otherwise, without the prior permission of Springer Publishing Company, Inc.

Springer Publishing Company, Inc.
11 West 42nd Street
New York, NY 10036

Acquisitions Editor: Sheri W. Sussman
Production Editor: Sara Yoo
Cover design by Joanne Honigman
Typeset by Daily Information Processing, Churchville, PA

06 07 08 09 10 / 5 4 3 2 1

Library of Congress Cataloging-in-Publication Data

Wainrib, Barbara Rubin.
    Healing crisis and trauma with mind, body, and spirit / Barbara Rubin Wainrib.
        p. ; cm.
    Includes bibliographical references and index.
    ISBN 0-8261-3245-6
    1. Post-traumatic stress disorder—Treatment. 2. Psychic trauma—Treatment. 3. Crisis intervention (Mental health services). I. Title.
    [DNLM: 1. Stress Disorders, Post-Traumatic—therapy.
    2. Counseling. 3. Crisis Intervention. 4. Disasters. 5. Life Change Events. 6. Violence—psychology. WM 170 W244h 2006]
    RC552.P67W32   2006
    616.85'21—dc22

                                                                    2005032352

Printed in the United States of America by Bang Printing.

*As always, this book is dedicated to the memory of my beloved
Grandma Ada—Ada Kaufman Berman, who taught me*

"Whatever you undertake, God will help you."

*It is also dedicated to the memory of the victims
of terrorism and trauma around the world,
and to all of those healers who work with the victims.*

To Doron X, who knows why!

*To my dear husband, Charles Wainrib,
who has survived a very difficult year.*

To my children, Jeannine, Andrew, and Rod Merl.

*And to my beloved granddaughter, Rachel Wainrib Friendly,
who begins her doctoral program in clinical psychology
at Clark University as I write this, and to whom I say,*

"Whatever you undertake, God will help you."

Contents

Preface

We live in a changed world, a world where the enemy is no longer in uniform on the other side of a trench. There is no longer an identified "war zone" and the "enemy" may be the innocent-looking person standing next to us. Clear boundaries and an assumption of safety no longer exist.

The enemy is in offices, in peaceful-looking aircraft that suddenly destroy whole buildings and thousands of innocent lives; the enemy is on buses and subways at rush hour. We can no longer differentiate between counselors and therapists, or crisis and trauma victims because all of us are potential victims of the latter and need the skills of the former. In addition, emerging changes in our weather system have turned our beloved "Mother Nature" into a terrifying villain. We simply can no longer know when, where, or how trauma will present itself, or when we may be called upon to help a myriad of innocent victims.

This book is written for those persons in the "helping professions." It is also written for those who have a sufficient understanding of psychology and a sufficient awareness of our current world and who want to gain some knowledge about being helpful. We now know that learning new skills to address the injuries incurred by sudden trauma and unpredictable lives is essential. For many years, I have been doing research about trauma. In addition to applying this research in my own practice, I have been teaching and supervising other therapists, as well as teaching graduate students at McGill University and post-graduates around the continent. These experiences have not only reinforced the importance of knowing theory, but of teaching it in hands-on fashion.

This book offers the educator and the practitioner training methods, exercises, and intervention techniques applicable to the gamut of experiences that we currently encounter. It also will introduce readers to newer concepts and their applications, such as role play, spirituality, the role of animals in healing, and the concept of forgiveness. Throughout the book, whether it is in those who represent the highly resilient or those who continue to struggle, a strengths perspective is emphasized. Finally, this book describes the "Phoenix Phenomenon," a concept I developed during the course of my teaching and practice, which articulates and illustrates an inherent ability to use resilience in the process of converting pain into growth.

I hope that this book will enrich the reader both professionally and personally and will provide new resources to renew our faith in this difficult and unpredictable world.

Acknowledgments

Those of you who have been my colleagues and students (as well as all of you who will read this book) know of a concept I created called the "Phoenix Phenomenon," which refers to the capacity for growth after crisis and about which you will read later in these pages. My initial publication of this concept was in 1972, and it continues to be valid, as you will see in chapter 6. This book, however, is, in itself, a "phoenix phenomenon." Without the support of Dr. Ursula Springer and Sheri Sussman of Springer Publishing Company, it would never have existed. A new creation arose from the ashes of a very painful situation, and I am deeply grateful to both of them for their responsiveness and their support.

Were it not for an important conversation with a special (unnameable!) friend, I may never have had that "Aha!" moment that showed me the direction I needed. (And I would not have gotten to that conversation were it not for his mother—so, yes, sometimes mothers do help!)

Although I have written and edited several books, this is the first time that I have totally flown solo. It definitely has both advantages and disadvantages, and I am very grateful to my family for their varied types of support. I am deeply indebted to my beloved daughter, Jeannine Wainrib, a multigifted young woman who moves gracefully from rearranging peoples' lives to editing and rearranging her mother's writings. And all of this is done in the midst of making a major life change herself, joining with Dr. Rod Merl, an equally caring and helpful soul.

For many years, we have been a family of dedicated Macintosh users, believers, and supporters. However, during this experience, I started to believe that Macintoshes were allergic to me. Not one but both of my otherwise trusty machines tested my faith and seemed to have rebelled against me. The final blow came when, dangerously close to my deadline, my "user-friendly" Mac moved itself into an otherwise unknown program (I think from Mars, but definitely not from Venus!). It refused to respond to my requests and eliminated rather important things! As always, I am deeply grateful to Charles, my husband of 54 years, who once again became the high-tech trauma responder. Having been together this long, we appreciate our different thinking patterns and languages, and our abilities to transfer skills when necessary! I hope that we will be able to continue this synchrony for many more years and for many more Macs and books. My son, Andrew, as always, provided comic relief, and my granddaughter, Rachel Wainrib Friendly, provided some drama as she applied to doctoral programs in clinical psychology. Yes, dear reader, she is currrently fulfilling her dream. So, despite the "Macintosh rebellion," the apples continue to fall close to the tree!

And last, but not in any way least, I am grateful to the peaceful, loving presence of Mello, a beautiful but seriously abused Labrador retriever that we saved from sure death at the SPCA a few years ago. When you read chapter 10, you will hear of her therapeutic role and understand my feelings!

We live in a world that seems to proliferate traumas, and wherever we look, there are emotional wounds that need healing. "Man's inhumanity to man" seems to be at an all-time high, unfortunately. Those of us in this field need to refresh hopes, beliefs, and knowledge regularly for themselves as well as for those they treat. My own hope is that while reading this book, you will have new learnings, or even a sudden "Aha" that will allow you to help heal some of the incredible numbers of wounded souls in our increasingly difficult world. Additionally, I hope it will refresh your own mind, body, and spirit and protect them from an overdose of pain.

BARBARA RUBIN WAINRIB, EdD
Montreal, Canada
April 2005

CHAPTER 1

Understanding Crisis Intervention and Trauma Response

INTRODUCTION:
REVIEW OF THE GENERAL CRISIS RESPONSE

The *General Crisis Response* is a concept that was developed during the writing of our previous book, *Crisis Intervention and Trauma Response: Theory and Practice* (Wainrib & Bloch, 1998). In it, we attempted to integrate the two concepts *life crisis* and *trauma.* We described life crisis as an experience that generally relates to more predictable experiences such as birth, illness, divorce, and so on. Trauma is generally sudden, drastic, and often life threatening. Examples of trauma are the London bombings, September 11, 2001 (9-11), rape; war; natural disasters; and others.

In our earlier book, we said that "As the world becomes more and more complex and varieties of both crisis and trauma seem to be taking on greater visibility on a regular basis, this concept itself takes on larger significance."

For the sake of simplicity, throughout the present book, the author will integrate the general crisis response and use the term trauma as all inclusive.

The material that you are about to read is an enlargement and update of the vast new knowledge that has been created in this field in the relatively short time since the 1998 book.

ACKNOWLEDGING TRAUMA

Most human beings who live in a relatively peaceful environment such as North America assume that they can face each day in a fairly predictable manner. We see outbreaks of wars and uprisings on our television news and

1

silently give thanks that we live in the comfort of safety. This reinforces our childhood belief that we will somehow be protected and secure. As adults, we assume the responsibility for our own safety and that of our offspring. We may know that our streets are not as safe as they once were, but our mental mechanism of denial is generally well functioning. When the evening news reports horror stories, they are rarely in our neighborhood, and we can, once again, reassure ourselves. We live with the subconscious knowledge that horror and trauma exist but assume that it cannot happen here. Denial is a great gift! Hence, it is not surprising that resistance to recognizing the realities of trauma has been exceptional. Trauma was simply something either relatively unknown or an experience that happened somewhere else. This is, however, no longer the case.

HISTORICAL BACKGROUND: MEN, WOMEN, AND TRAUMA

Although a literature on the subject of crisis intervention has existed for over 50 years, trauma response, like psychology itself, has a long past and a short history. As we look back with a current perspective to the manner in which responses to traumatic events were perceived and how trauma itself was defined, it is not surprising to see that much of this information was based on images of gender stereotypes. During the First World War, men were supposed to "act like men" and have a "stiff upper lip." When, as a result of the horrors of war, they developed symptoms of shell shock or battle fatigue, they were considered unmanly. As Judith Lewis Herman, in her beautiful book, *Trauma and Recovery* (1992), describes it,

> [In the first World War] under conditions of unremitting exposure to the horrors of trench warfare, men began to break down in shocking numbers, confined and rendered helpless, subjected to constant threat of annihilation, they screamed and wept uncontrollably. They froze and could not move . . . became mute and unresponsive. One typical response was to strap the patient into a chair, apply electrical shocks to his throat, and, as the shocks were being applied to say "Remember you must behave as the hero I expect you to be. . . . A man who has gone through so many battles should have better control of himself."

During the Korean War, for the first time, clinicians provided frontline treatment for psychiatric breakdowns, returning the soldiers to battle as soon as possible afterward. However, when the same approach was attempted during the Vietnam era, very few combatants sought help. (Instead, the widespread use of marijuana and heroin apparently allowed them to complete their year of combat without breakdowns). There was yet no official traumatic-stress diagnosis, and the Veteran's Administration (VA) assumed that any psychiatric problem occurring more than 1 year after discharge could not be related to military service. However, after the soldiers returned to stateside, more than 50% began breaking down.

There was, however, considerable controversy about the responsibility for these veterans. Hence, it is not surprising that resistance to recognizing the realities of trauma was impressive. In 1978, my colleague, Charles Figley, a Vietnam veteran himself, published *Stress Disorders Among Vietnam Veterans,* which was the first acknowledgement of symptoms in this cohort.

After decades of sustaining these attitudes, pressure by groups such as the Vietnam Veterans Against the War and people like Charles Figley and Robert Jay Lifton finally led, in 1980, to the American Psychiatric Association's recognition of the significance of psychological trauma and addition of a new disorder category, posttraumatic stress disorder (PTSD), was included in the *Diagnostic and Statistical Manual of Mental Disorders IV (DSM IV)*. Its description follows:

309.81 Posttraumatic Stress Disorder
A. The person has been exposed to a traumatic event in which both of the following were present:
   (1) the person experienced, witnessed, or was confronted with an event or events that involved actual or threatened death or serious injury, or a threat to the physical integrity of self or others
   (2) the person's response involved intense fear, helplessness, or horror. Note In children, this may be expressed instead by disorganized or agitated behavior
B. The traumatic event is persistently reexperienced in one (or more) of the following ways:
   (1) recurrent and intrusive distressing recollections of the event, including images, thoughts or perceptions. Note: In young children, repetitive play may occur in which the themes or aspects of the trauma are expressed.
   (2) recurrent distressing dreams of the event. Note: In children, there may be frightening dreams without recognizable content.
   (3) acting or feeling as if the traumatic event were recurring (includes a sense of reliving the experience, illusions. Hallucinations and dissociative flashback episodes, including those that occur on awakening or when intoxicated).
   (4) intense psychological distress at exposure to internal or external cues that symbolize or resemble an aspect of the traumatic event.
   (5) physiological reactivity on exposure to internal or external cues that symbolize or resemble an aspect of the traumatic event.

C. Persistent avoidance of stimuli associated with the trauma and numbing of general responsiveness (not present before the trauma), as indicated by three (or more) of the following:
  (1) efforts to avoid thoughts, feelings, or conversations associated
      with the trauma
  (2) efforts to avoid activities, places, or people that arouse recollec-
      tions of the trauma
  (3) inability to recall an important aspect of the trauma
  (4) markedly diminished interest or participation in significant activities
  (5) feeling of detachment or estrangement from others
  (6) restricted range of affect (e.g., unable to have loving feelings)
  (7) sense of a foreshortened future (e.g., does not expect to have a
      career, marriage, children, or a normal life span)
D. Persistent symptoms of increased arousal (not present before the
trauma), as indicated by two (or more) of the following:
  (1) difficulty falling or staying asleep
  (2) irritability or outbursts of anger
  (3) difficulty concentrating
  (4) hypervigilance
  (5) exaggerated startle response
E. Duration of the disturbance (symptoms in Criteria B, C, and D) is
more than 1 month.
F. The disturbance causes clinically significant distress or impairment in
social, occupational or other important areas of functioning.

Specify if:
Acute: if duration of symptoms is less than 3 months
Chronic: if duration of symptoms is 3 months or more

Specify if:
With Delayed Onset: if onset of symptoms is at least 6 months after the
stressor

Women fared no better. Many of us are familiar with Jeffrey Moossaieff
Masson's book, *The Assault on Truth* (1998), in which the author reveals
Freud's dismissal of women's early memories of sexual abuse as "fantasy"
and therefore considers these memories to be insignificant. Innumerable
women have suffered not only the pain and trauma of childhood sexual
abuse, but the disbelief of those they sought to help them. Herman (1992)
tells us the following:

> For most of the twentieth century, it was the study of combat veterans
> that led to the body of knowledge about traumatic disorders. Not until
> the women's liberation movement in the 1970s was it recognized that
> the most common posttraumatic disorders are those not of men in war
> but of women in civilian life. . . . Women were silenced by fear and
> shame and the silence gave license to every form of sexual and domes-
> tic exploitation.

As the Women's Movement encouraged women to join together and speak out, which led to the creation of consciousness-raising groups, many of the horrors of the reality of their lives surfaced. In the 1970s, rape centers were set up, research was initiated, and women's needs began to be recognized. In so doing, many of the "secrets" of their own sexual traumas were finally revealed and validated. My colleague and friend, Dr. Lenore Walker, created and wrote poignantly about the condition known as the Battered-Woman Syndrome, and shelters for women who were abused by their spouses started to be created.

Herman (1992) adds the following:

> Psychological trauma is the affliction of the powerless. At the moment of trauma, the victim is rendered helpless by overwhelming force. When the force is of nature we speak of disasters. When the force is human beings, we speak of atrocities. Traumatic events overwhelm the ordinary systems of care that give people a sense of control, connections, and meaning.

MASS TRAUMAS

Although individual trauma has existed throughout history, mass trauma, such as that seen in war, terrorism, and epidemics, is considerably less frequent. Nevertheless, research on mass trauma has indicated that there have been instances of it worldwide since biblical times and perhaps even before. While the United States prefers to feel that it has rarely been associated with this experience, one must remember the country's roots. The historical facts of the forceful elimination and constraint of many Native Americans as well as the use of slavery in the South both qualify for this definition.

More recent mass trauma experiences, such as earlier terrorist activities in both New York City (1993) and Oklahoma City (1995), were rare on our continent. Residents of the United States, having had the privilege of living in a relatively protected world until that time, made the possibility of the creation of a mass trauma such as that which we experienced on 9-11 seem unrealistic. Trauma created by international terrorism has, however, been a part of our world for decades. Like many of us, I have had friends, relatives, colleagues, patients, and students in my McGill University courses who have described terrifying personal and familial experiences in some of the more oppressive countries from which they migrated. There are, of course, memories of the holocausts that took place both in Europe as well as in Rwanda. One of the more common responses to witnessing mass trauma in other people's countries is, however, a sense of denial.

Despite what we have seen and heard from refugees fleeing countries that have experienced mass trauma, we still try to believe that "this cannot happen here." It is only since 9-11 that we (North Americans) have recognized the degree of our personal vulnerability and the loss of our innocence. Our previously protected space has now been violated, our inner sense of invulnerability has been challenged, and our perception of the world has changed. Reflecting the impact of this dramatic change, the word trauma has become a household word.

This book deals with a world that has changed, a world in which strategies that were normally used to maintain security can no longer help us. Thinking back to that terrible day of 9-11 will give us a sense of what trauma can feel like, whether we experienced it personally or whether we identified with some of the families and friends of victims that we saw on the screen. It will help us to understand the meaning and experience of crisis and trauma as well as to look at new strategies that each of us may have considered but perhaps have not applied to times of change and difficulty.

I will not limit our concept of trauma to those threats that are external. Instead, I will respect the responses of the body and incorporate the internal trauma of life-threatening illnesses. Trauma and health are interactive, as we will see in chapter 5. Trauma in itself can create many significant bodily reactions. Conversely, illness, particularly serious illness, can create traumatic responses.

I will also go beyond that to find ways in which three essential modalities—body, mind, and spirit—can be called upon to help ourselves, our friends, our families, our colleagues, and our clients heal in these times when trauma is no longer a stranger but can reappear at any time and in any place. More than anything else, we need to remember the following powerful words of Ernest Hemingway: "The world breaks everyone . . . and afterward, some are strong at the broken places." Learning how to not only survive but to *use* life crisis and trauma is the mission of this book. Its goal is to teach how to help ourselves, our students, our clients, and our loved ones to grow strong at the broken places.

REFERENCES

Figley, C. (1978). *Stress disorders among Vietnam veterans: Theory, research and treatment*. New York: Brunner Mazel.

Herman, J. L. (1992). *Trauma and recovery*. New York: Basic Books.

Masson, J. M. (1998). *The assault on truth: Freud's suppression of the seduction theory*. New York: Pocket Books.

CHAPTER 2

Understanding Trauma and Its Impact

Experiencing trauma is an essential part of being human: History is written in blood.

—B. Van der Kolk and colleagues (1996)

SEPTEMBER 11, 2001: THE PSYCHOLOGICAL EXPERIENCE—REACTION AND RESPONSE

There is probably not a soul in North America or perhaps in the world who will ever forget September 11, 2001 (9-11). It was a day that, for many of us, changed our view of our world, our image of security, and our expectations of the future. For almost all of us, it was a marker event, a life crisis. For many, however, it was also a trauma. We each have a memory of it engraved into our minds, hearts and souls, and memory banks.

What Jeffery Kauffman refers to as the "loss of our assumptive world," the world previously experienced as normal or predictable (Kauffman, 2002), was altered permanently for us on 9-11.

ARE WE ALL VICTIMS?

There is a very significant statement engraved on the arches of the memorial built for the April 19, 1995, terrorist bombing in Oklahoma City. At that time, this destructive act was the worst act of terrorism perpetrated in the United States.

The text of the monument says, "To those who were killed, those who survived, and those whose lives changed forever." It is the equivalent for the victims of 9-11.

Some of us have sustained personal losses or are connected to direct survivors, some of us worked directly with survivors and absorbed their experiences, and all of our lives have changed forever. We need to be able to make rational sense of this new world, both for ourselves and for our clients and patients. In order to do that, we must each understand our own reactions and their meaning.

Let us look at my reactions, one who was geographically distant from the events of 9-11, as well as the reactions of some of my colleagues who were right there. "I walked out of my office in Montreal with my 8 AM patient, her session concluded. I was surprised to see my husband in the corridor. Although we work in the same area, we rarely see each other during the day. As soon as my client left, he rushed over and said "Barbara, they've bombed the World Trade Center!" I could not believe what I heard, and I asked him to repeat it several times as I tried to comprehend it. My next reaction was "How could they get bombs on a commercial airplane?" and then, before he had a chance to answer, I said, *This does not happen in North America,"* almost as if it were some kind of mantra of belief that I had to cling to in the face of overwhelming emotion, some magical way in which I tried to undo the reality.

At the physical level, I experienced a sense of shivering as the overwhelming fear started to break through. Then came a sense of terror as I realized the absolute horror of it. My attempts to connect with friends, family, and loved ones in New York and in other major American cities were mostly unsuccessful.

This is how Kathleen Nader (2001), a social worker, described her reaction in *Gift From Within:*

> We have been inundated with painful images and stories. Concerns such as those regarding the dead, the injured (physically and/or emotionally), future vulnerability, the need to strike back, business losses, costs of restoration and protection, and more fill our thoughts and are regularly discussed in the media. The stresses have been unrelenting. The danger has not ceased. We wonder about the threat of another terrorist act. In New York there is continued danger from building debris, rescuer overwork, and other aspects of the cleanup process. For a long time, we hoped that people remained alive under the debris.

Some of my colleagues have shared their experiences with me. These include Dr. Ken Pope, who wrote:

It's hard for me to think of any colleague I've spent time with in person or on the phone who hasn't been knocked way off balance by the 9-11 mass murders and all that has followed. The sudden, massive loss of human life and all that it means have been so hard to take in and be with, so hard for the heart to hold.

He then described how this experience challenged the physical and psychological resources even of those who are skilled and conscientious about their self-care. "The result is everything from headaches, insomnia, confusion, memory problems, intrusive images to the full range of PTSD, depression, and almost unendurable distress" (Personal communication, 2003).

Dr. Sandra Haber, a colleague who lives and practices in New York City, starts her reminiscence: "My office is located in upper midtown on the island of Manhattan. At 9:20 my patient arrives and tells me that a plane has hit the World Trade Center. We both lament this unfortunate accident and the probable loss of life, but go on with our session." She continued, "After the session, I retrieve my messages. The first is from my husband, who says something about the World Trade Center being bombed. My machine cut him off in the middle. . . . The second from a patient who . . . commutes from New Jersey . . . saying that the tunnel was closed . . . and something terrible had happened in lower Manhattan. . . . I call my husband and get more information. I'm upset, but, to his chagrin, I don't quite get it. I listen to my radio and begin to see the enormity of the situation." She then finds a neighbor with a TV set. "The young man and I watch as the Trade Center crumbles."

> Back in my office, the phone rings, and my 13-year-old daughter bursts into tears when she hears my voice. . . . She didn't know where I worked relative to the World Trade Center. I think her tears made the event real for me. I know I was more upset than I realized, because I chose to walk down the 21 flights of stairs instead of taking the elevator. In retrospect, my automatic pilot had kicked in.

UNDERSTANDING REACTIONS

Dr. Haber's reactions started with denial. She was not quite getting it when her husband tried to describe the reality of the situation to her. This was followed by an emotional breakthrough with her child, causing the denial and rationalization aspect of her reactions to be altered. However, the numbness remained as she walked down 21 flights of stairs instead of taking the elevator. Her automatic pilot had indeed kicked in.

YOUR REACTION

Although considerable time has passed since the initial impact of 9-11, experiences such as these often stay deeply engraved on our psyches. Can you recall, now, after time has passed, what kinds of reactions you had on that fateful morning? Try to bring to mind the following:

- Where were you when you heard of the attack?
- What did you think?
- What did you feel emotionally?
- What was happening in your body?

If you really stay in touch with your reactions as we take you back to that horrible experience, you will have some indication of your own initial reaction, at the cognitive, behavioral, and affective level, to this crisis or trauma.

A typical theme found in most people's reactions is that they all carry within them a core of denial. An almost immediate reaction to any situation which will abruptly change your life is the response of denial: This is not happening—make it not happen! Or, in this case, this does not happen here in my country or to me. In a previous work, we described this feeling as follows:

> There is the sense within each of us that we walk around in the world in a protected magic bubble, one that keeps our world relatively stable and predictable. It keeps the terrifying things, the unpredictable things, the life-disrupting things, away from us. Yes, we hurt, we fear, we cry (Wainrib, in Wainrib & Bloch, 1998).

For most of us, the really terrible things in the world—terrorism, accidents, life-threatening illness, disasters—do not invade our bubble of invisible invincibility. They happen to other people, but not to us. If or when they do invade our personal magic bubble, they bring about a complete reappraisal of our selves, our life, and our way of being in the world. A reappraisal of this magnitude is, at best, difficult for us to fathom. When life presents us with an opportunity to reassess ourselves under the most comfortable of situations, it is painful, time-consuming, and confusing. When this reassessment and pressure to change erupts upon our consciousness at a time when all or many of our stabilities have been threatened, it is that much more so. Hence, the reaction of "they cannot get a bomb on board an airplane," which, in effect, says: "Kill the messenger."

This foolish person is making an impossibly ridiculous mistake, and if I can just eliminate the messenger bearing that mistake, it will all disappear, and my life will go on as before.

A disaster of the magnitude of 9-11 is so enormous that it feeds our sense of disbelief. Most of us have been privileged to live in relatively stable environments. We hear about terrible things, but essentially, we feel protected. The events of 9-11, tore into our belief in a protected world and made us all subject to a vulnerability that was previously denied or nonexistent.

The second half of this reaction is,

> Make it yesterday: Make this change be undone and let my life go on as it did before this terrible thing happened. The "Stop Today—Make It Yesterday" theme is one we will encounter a great deal in dealing with people in crisis. Hence the two themes of denial (this is not happening) and undoing (make this not have happened) are defensive reactions that many people will try to use in any life crisis or trauma (Wainrib, in Wainrib & Bloch, 1998).

UNDERSTANDING TRAUMA

Judith Lewis Herman (1992), a gifted specialist in the trauma area, tells us

> Traumatic events are extraordinary, not because they occur rarely, but rather because they overwhelm the ordinary adaptations to life. Unlike commonplace misfortunes, traumatic events generally involve threats to life or bodily integrity, or a close personal encounter with death. They confront human beings with the extremities of helplessness and terror, and evoke the responses of catastrophe. The common denominator of trauma is a feeling of intense fear, helplessness, loss of control and threat annihilation (p. 33).

Other specialists in this field define psychological trauma. Trauma occurs when

1. The individual's ability to integrate his or her emotional experience is overwhelmed.
2. The individual experiences (subjectively) a threat to life, bodily integrity, or sanity.

The International Society for Traumatic Stress Studies (ISTSS) tells us that

Traumatic events are shocking and emotionally overwhelming situations. It is natural for people who experience or witness them to have many reactions. Some of these are intense fear, horror, numbness, or helplessness. These events might involve actual or threatened death, serious injury, or sexual or other physical assault.

They can be one-time occurrences, such as a natural disaster, house fire, violent crime, or airplane accident, or they can be ongoing, repeated, and relentless, as is often the case in combat or war. Child abuse and neglect and other forms of domestic violence are additional examples of this. Most often, trauma is accompanied by many losses. Unfortunately, traumatic events are quite common.

Reactions to traumatic events vary considerably, ranging from relatively mild, creating minor disruptions in the person's life, to severe and debilitating. It is very common for people to experience anxiety, terror, shock, and upset, as well as emotional numbness and personal or social disconnection. People often cannot remember significant parts of what happened, yet may be plagued by parts of memories that return in physical and psychological flashbacks. Nightmares of the traumatic event are common, as are depression, irritability, sleep disturbance dissociation, and feeling jumpy (ISTSS, 2003).

In your work with traumatized populations, you may encounter all of the experiences described above or perhaps only a few. None of us walk lockstep through life, and this concept of uniqueness in each individual is writ large in our work with trauma victims. Experiences that create trauma are contrary to our expectations of normal human life, and thus, create reactions of shock, disbelief, incredibility, and, in some cases, a total change of our perception of the world.

Immediately after the occurrence of the trauma, some clients may feel the need to have a comforting listener validate their experience. Others may prefer to be alone or to be with familiar caring friends or relatives. Many, however, will be unable to discuss the experience. Traumatic events can cause severe psychological reactions that can manifest themselves at anytime. For example, a young woman of my acquaintance was in the World Trade Center just as the second plane hit. Fortunately, she was on the ground floor and managed to escape. As of this writing, she has not yet been able to discuss her experience, and she rejects attempts of loved ones and helping professionals to evoke her memories.

For some, such as many war veterans, the traumatic event remains to haunt them throughout their lifetime. Dr. Lisa Lewis (1998), director of neuropsychological services at the Menninger Clinic writes:

None of us wants to believe we will ever fall victim to assault, damaging industrial or motor vehicle accidents, or horrific natural disasters that threaten to shatter our bodies, our lives, and our fundamental relationships. Yet, statistics indicate that the majority of us will have such an experience in our lifetimes.

When our tragedies are met with understanding and compassionate responses from others, our suffering is alleviated or even entirely eliminated, and some few of us will even grow from the experience. . . . In this sense, Nietzsche was right in saying that whatever doesn't kill me will make me stronger (Foreword).

VICARIOUS TRAUMATIZATION

All of those people whose lives are touched by a traumatic experience become to one extent or another secondary or vicarious victims. The impact on them can vary tremendously, but should not be overlooked nor ignored. It is important to include these people in your contact both at trauma sites a well as in the larger population. For example, a year after the 9-11 disaster, family members of victims were invited back to Ground Zero for a very moving ceremony. The ceremony, however, was not really enough to deal with their pain. A colleague of ours who participated in it reported that many of the participants seemed to want a piece of the ground, or a plant, or something that concretely represented a grave site for their beloved, lost family members. When my colleague handed them tissues personally, rather than having them pick up their own, they were deeply moved by the important and often overlooked human touch. These were just some small but important external expressions of their experience. In a later chapter, we will devote more time to a description of the impact of trauma not only on loved ones but also on the helpers who work with them.

In my previous book (Wainrib & Bloch, 1998), I described the "Phoenix Phenomenon" as follows:

> Our own experiences with the lives of clients, as well as our own life, has led us to the concept of the Phoenix Phenomenon, which is the ultimate goal of empowerment. The Phoenix, as you may recall, was a mythic bird that had the capacity to resurrect itself, to rise, at it were, from its own ashes. Our work has shown that the impact of life crisis or trauma can provoke either a positive or negative response which has the potential for change in the direction of one's life.

The 9-11 experience, horrible as it was, had a similar impact on some people. My colleague, Dr. Pat Pitta, found that the impact of 9-11 was, in effect a "Phoenix Phenomenon" for her. The 9-11 experience created her own personal life reassessment. Now, in addition to her busy psychotherapy practice, she is also a student in the ministry (Pitta, personal communication, 2001).

Dr. Ken Pope, quoted earlier, tells us that

one of most striking aspects [of 9-11] has been the great number of colleagues for whom these events (and the insomnia, nightmares, forgetfulness, etc., that have accompanied them) have served as transformative experiences. A wake-up call or reminder that they have not been using whatever time they have in the ways that matter most to them. They've started saying things to loved ones, and being different toward loved ones (and "liked ones," too—and perhaps even "unliked ones"). They feel as if they had been lulled to sleep by the habitual nature of what they'd been doing, or the seeming lack of options, or the constant pressures and overcrowded schedules and showers of worries (often about things that, in retrospect, seem not very important), and had been drifting (or running in place) through their lives. They use their time differently and go about what they do with a different approach. In some cases their priorities change profoundly.

Dr. Russ Newman (2002), an executive of the American Psychological Association, quotes Victor Frankl from *Man's Search for Meaning* (Frankl, 1963):

Even the helpless victim of a hopeless situation, facing a fact he can not change may rise above himself, may grow beyond himself, he may turn personal tragedy into triumph, and turn his predicament into a human achievement.

Newman continues and tells us:

As a part of the role psychologists must play following this tragedy we must act as guides for the psychological journey of our country to find meaning in these events. We must use our knowledge, our research and our clinical skill to help turn personal tragedy into triumph and to turn our predicament into a human achievement. . . . We must put aside our personal and professional differences so that we do not shirk this responsibility or squander this opportunity. I am confident our profession will rise to this occasion. Many are counting on us.

You may find that referring to these reactions will be of help in understanding your own reactions as well as those of your clients. For many of us, our initial reaction to 9-11 was one of numbing and disbelief. Then the feelings started flooding our psyches. Bruce Hiley-Young, a trauma specialist, puts it well when he says, "Trauma and disaster rupture the individual and collective effort to understand, organize, preserve, sustain and make meaning of life." And so it does.

Many of us may have had a variety of symptoms as a result of this experience. We may have had sleep disturbances, unexpected anger and irritability, concentration difficulties, restlessness, social withdrawal, and many other otherwise strange reactions. Depending upon our own individual, familial, and cultural histories of previous traumas, these symptoms may have been mild or severe; they may have stayed rooted in this moment or flashed us back to other personal horrors. What we needed at that moment was a sense of a safe place, either within ourselves or in the outside world, and a good support network of people who were able talk, listen, and understand.

Pyszczynski, Solomon, and Greenberg (2002) describe a concept that they call terror management, which has relevance here. It includes the concept that

> at the most fundamental level, cultures allow people to control the ever-present potential terror of death by convincing them that they are beings of enduring significance living in a meaningful reality. . . . [Attacks such as 9-11] disrupt our normal means of managing our natural terror and, in so doing, threatened to undermine our psychological equanimity necessary for people to function effectively on a daily basis. . . . The juxtaposition of a biological predisposition toward self-preservation that human beings share with all forms of life with the uniquely human awareness of the inevitability of death gives rise to potentially overwhelming terror (p. 135).

SECONDARY VICTIMS

All of those people whose lives are touched by a traumatic experience become to one extent or another "secondary" or "vicarious" victims. The impact on them can vary tremendously but should not be overlooked nor ignored. It is important to include these people in your contact, both at trauma sites as well as in the larger population.

Part of the process of working through a traumatic experience calls into question basic beliefs the individual holds about life. A number of authors have described one central belief as that of a "just world." A crisis or trauma disrupts the bedrock of a belief in a just world. How persons respond, in the long run, depends on how they perceive their newly configured world and their place in it, especially their relationship to others.

Possible Obstacles to Help-Seeking After Trauma

It may seem surprising to some of us in the helping professions that there are times when we are surprised at the small number of people who seem to need our help immediately following a traumatic experience. The National Center for PTSD has analyzed this issue and have prepared this very helpful fact sheet: "Several studies have pointed out that following a terrorist event such as the Oklahoma City bombing, many of those in closest proximity to the disaster do not believe they need help, and will not seek out services, despite reporting significant emotional distress" (Meyer, 1991; Sprang, 2000). Sprang lists several potential reasons for this. These include a feeling that one is better off; pride, that is, a feeling that distress indicates weakness; difficulty in acknowledging that services they received are mental health related. Sprang has found that "Many individuals are more apt to seek informal support from family and friends, which may not be sufficient to prevent long-term distress in some."

North and colleagues (1999) found in a study of survivors of the Oklahoma City bombing that nearly half of those who had direct exposure had an "active post-disaster psychiatric disorder, with PTSD being diagnosed in $^1/_3$ of the respondents." Meyer (1991) teaches us that "Major Depression was the most commonly associated disorder. . . . Symptom onset of PTSD was rather immediate, usually within one or two days, and few other cases developed after the first month."

The Phenomenon of Loss in a Community

The 9-11 disaster highlighted an entire community's experience of the phenomenon of loss. Writer Garry Cooper reported in the *Psychotherapy Networker* (2002, p. 13) on a national survey conducted by the *New England Journal of Medicine* between September 14 and 16, 2001. In it, respondents were asked to rate their experience of various symptoms of anxiety such as disturbing memories, difficulty concentrating, sleeping problems and increased irritability, on a scale of one to five. Forty-four percent rated their experience of at least one of the symptoms as "substantial," and 46% rated their experience of at least one symptom as "moderate." Adults also reported that 35% of their children were suffering from elevated stress levels. In the same article, commenting on the impact of the anthrax scare that came shortly on the heels of 9-11, British psychologist Simon Wessley, writing in the October 20 issue of the *British Medical Journal,* said "The general elevation of malaise, fear and anxiety may remain high for years, exacerbating preexisting psychiatric disorders and further heightening the risks of mass sociogenic illness" (Wessley, 2001).

Risk Factors

Let us look at some of the elements that determine an individual's response to trauma. Norris, Byrne, Diaz, and Kaniasty (2001) have prepared a review of the empirical literature of risk factors for adverse outcomes in natural and human-caused disasters. Their work differentiates between predisaster, disaster, within-disaster, and postdisaster factors. The findings of Norris and colleagues (2001) that are most pertinent to my work follow.

Predisaster Factors

Regardless of the method of data collection, predisaster symptoms were almost always among the best (if not the best) predictors of postdisaster symptoms.

Of the predisaster factors, the following were most significant. Gender influenced postdisaster outcomes in 45 samples, as follows: In 42 (93%) of 45 samples, women or girls were affected more adversely by disasters than were men or boys. Panel studies indicated that psychological effects were not only stronger among women but more lasting as well.

Age and Experience

One of the most interesting findings of Norris and colleagues is that "older adults were at greater risk than were other adults in only 2 (14%) of the 14 adult samples. Rather than as an at-risk group, older adults might be viewed as a resource for disaster stricken communities." This is a crucial piece of information, and I suspect it is a surprise to many readers. As you will see, it creates an unexpected new well of potential helpers. However, they warn us that "in every American sample where middle-aged adults were differentiated from older and younger adults, they were most adversely affected." In a later chapter, I will discuss the impact of earlier experiences on older adults. We can speculate from these findings that middle age has its own potential for crisis and turmoil, whereas getting through that to "maturity" is a value in itself.

"People who have experienced disasters previously show higher levels of hazard preparedness and are more likely to evacuate when authorities suggest they do." However, it was noted that "professionalism and training increase the resilience of recovery workers, although past trauma per se does not."

All of the following have been found, at least in some studies, to predict adverse outcomes among survivors:

- Bereavement
- Injury to self or another family member
- Life threat
- Panic or similar emotions during the disaster
- Horror
- Separation from family (especially among youth)
- Extensive loss of property
- Relocation or displacement.

As the number of these stressors increased, the likelihood of psychological impairment increased. In general, injury and life threat were most predictive of long-term adverse consequences, especially PTSD.

Postdisaster Factors

Both life-event stress (discrete changes) and chronic stress were strong predictors of survivors' health outcomes. Moreover, stability and change in psychological symptoms were largely explained by stability and change in stress and resources. Some research suggests that the long-term effects of acute stressors (the individual-level aspects of exposure outlined above) on psychological distress operate through their effects on chronic stressors, such as marital stress, financial stress, and ecological stress.

Attention needs to be paid to stress levels in stricken communities long after the disaster has happened and passed.

A substantial amount of research pertinent to understanding risk factors for adverse outcomes has been published over the past 20 years. The research base is larger and more consistent for adults than it is for youth. Even for adults, more research on many of these topics would be quite useful and could eventually change the weight of the evidence. Nonetheless, at present, the literature reviewed yields the following conclusions:

An adult's risk will increase linearly along with the number of these factors that are present (Norris, Byrne, Diaz, & Kaniasty, 2001):

- Female gender
- Age in the middle years of 40 to 60
- Little previous experience or relevant training

REFERENCES

Cooper, G. (2002, January–February). *Psychotherapy Networker, 13.*

Frankl, V., Man's search for meaning. (Quoted in Newman, R., January 2002). *APA Monitor, 3,* 1.

Herman, J. L. (1992). *Trauma and recovery* (pp. 23, 33, 60). New York: Basic Books.

Hiley-Young, B. (1992). Traumatic reactivation and treatment: Integrated case examples. *Journal of Traumatic Stress, 5,* National Center for Traumatic Stress Disorder, 545–555.

International Society for Traumatic Stress Studies. (2003). *Stress Points.*

Kauffman, J. (2002). *Loss of our assumptive world.* Oxford, England: Brunner-Routledge.

Lewis, L. (1998). Forward to *Shocks to the system.* New York: Norton.

Meyer. (1991). *Mental health intervention for disasters: A National Center for PTSD fact sheet.*

Nader, K. (2001). Supplemental article to terrorism: September 11, 2001, trauma, grief and recovery. In J. Boaz, *Gift from within.*

Newman, R. (2002, January). Man's search for meaning. *APA Monitor, 2, 32*(1), 33.

Norris, F. H., Byrne, C. M., Diaz, E., & Kaniasty, K. (2001). *The range, magnitude, and duration of effects of natural and human-caused disasters: A review of the empirical literature.* Boston: National Center for PTSD.

North, Tivis, L., & McMillen, J. C. (1999). *Disasters and substance abuse or dependence: A fact sheet from the National Center for PTSD.*

Pyszczynski, T., Solomon, S., & Greenberg, J. (2003). *In the wake of 9-11—The psychology of terror.* Washington, DC: APA Books.

Sprang, G. (2000). Coping strategies and traumatic stress symptomatology following the Oklahoma City bombing. *Social Work and Social Sciences Review, 8*(2), 207–218.

Van der Kolk, B., McFarlane, A., & Weisaeth, L. (Eds.). (1996). *Traumatic stress: The effects of overwhelming experience on mind, body and society.* New York: Guilford Press.

Wainrib, B., & Bloch, E. (1998). *Crisis intervention and trauma response: Theory and practice.* New York: Springer Publishing Co.

Wessley, S. (2001). Implications for terror attacks. *British Medical Journal, (10),* 20.

CHAPTER 3

Mass Trauma: Past and Present

Everyone suffers. In times of war or calamity or natural disaster everyone suffers together. Yet no matter how far the dark ripples of pain might spread, suffering is always individual.

—Deepak Chopra (2002)

THE IMPACT OF MASS TRAUMA

Recovering from mass psychological trauma depends in part on people's ability to make sense of their experience. In order to do that, they need to answer questions such as, "Why did this happen to me, all of my loved ones, and my friends? Why did this happen to my community?" and "How can I be sure that I will be protected in the future?" "Who will protect me?" "Is there any safe place?" "Must I leave my community and my home to be safe?"

AFRICAN GENOCIDE

As many of us know, Rwanda, suffered a disastrous experience of mass killing and genocide within its borders. A mass genocide was imposed on the Tutsis by the Hutus. The genocide produced staggering statistics that indicate its enormity in terms of cope and process. It created an initial population displacement of 1.7 million Hutus fearing reprisals; left 400,000 widows; 500,000 orphans; and 130,000 imprisoned on suspicion of committing acts of genocide. The country's fledgling judicial system was all but destroyed in terms of personnel and infrastructure by the spring of 1994. The judiciary was a primary target during the genocide that eliminated 244 out of a precious 750 judges, with many survivors fleeing into exile. As late as 1997, the courts in Rwanda were left to function with only 50 lawyers and a notable absence of infrastructure and administration, specifically courts of appeal" (Tiemessen, 2004). Anyone who is reading this book is presumably engaged in some way with traumatic and posttraumatic experiences. Whether you are about to go into the world of healing trauma, are just studying it, or are an "old hand" at it, take a moment, if you would, to digest these statistics and try to imagine some way in which you would be able to heal people under these circumstances!

THE GACACA PROCESS

"Gacaca" (pronounced *Ga-cha-cha*) means "community justice." The word itself actually means "judgment on the grass." "It was used in its colonial form to moderate disputes concerning land use and rights, cattle, marriage, inheritance rights, loans, damage to properties caused by one of the parties or animals, and petty theft" (Werchick, quoted in Tiemessen, 2004). Gacaca was intended to "sanction the violation of rules that are shared by the community, with the sole objective of reconciliation" through restoring harmony and social order and reintegration of the person who was the source of the disorder (Organization for African Unity, quoted in Tiemessen).

It was felt by psychologists Pearlman and Staub (2002) that the purposes of the Gacaca process—that is, justice, healing, and reconciliation—might be advanced if people had ways of understanding how genocide can come about. In the Gacaca, 250,000 people elected from the general population acted as judges, in groups of 19, in over 10,000 locations around Rwanda. In addition, understanding psychological trauma and healing was hoped to minimize the retraumatization that may have occurred as a result of the Gacaca hearings in 1994. Tiemessen reports the following in the *Journal of African Studies* (2004):

> The epicenter of post-genocide Rwanda society and politics has been the need for reconciliation to assuage and end a culture of impunity. . . .

Unfortunately, as of August 2005, the goals of Gacaca have not been met. Gacaca was indeed a valiant approach to healing, using an age-old technique to deal with current problems. Many of us who have heard about it in North America were impressed with its applicability and looked at it as a potential healing process for mass trauma. Tiemessen (2004) informs us that Gacaca represents a model of restorative justice because it focuses on the healing of victims and perpetrators, confessions, plea bargains, and reintegration.

Tiemessen's study (2004) indicates that "the principles and process of these courts hoped to mitigate the (previous failures . . . and sought) to punish or reintegrate over hundreds and thousands of genocide suspects. . . . However, the revelations that Gacaca is reconciliatory justice does not preclude its potential for inciting ethnic rivalry."

Likewise, the prevention of genocide must include healing from past psychological wounds (Staub, 1998). A psychoeducational program that provided the two elements of psychosocial support and a conceptual framework could make an important impact.

Though they speak the same language, Hutus and Tutsis rarely mix, despite efforts made by some church leaders and community organizations to get them together. "The wounds of 1994 are still too fresh to heal" (Heinrich, 2005). Old attitudes linger.

TEN YEARS LATER

Now, more than 10 years later, despite an official ending to the massacre, little has changed in the hearts, minds and feelings of the groups. Many no longer reside in their homeland, and Canada has become a safe haven to a large number of displaced Rwandans. For both Tutsis and Hutus, the pain lingers, and with the pain, there is the distrust of the opposite group. Part of the problem is each group's ignorance of the other.

> The Tutsis claim that Rwanda has every right to secure its borders and for Hutus the conflict is seen as revenge, pure and simple. Rwanda Tutsis are still seen as using their moral advantage as victims of an African holocaust to wage war, by proxy or otherwise, on a larger neighbor.

As in all disputes, neither side is totally right nor wrong. Yet the blame continues to be attributed, and the diaspora is not immune to its effects.

The recent release of a film (Hotel Rwanda) has elicited much interest in both groups, and it may very well reawaken some of the pain, even as it strives to heal.

Creating Hope

One interesting project, which was presented at the recent meeting of the International Society for Traumatic Stress Studies, is called Nah We Yone, Inc., Creating Hope Support and Safety Out of Chaos. They tell us that

> The trauma and chaos created by war has forced numerous Africans to flee their countries of origin. Those seeking refuge are forced to manage the sequelae of their past traumas, while coping with the cultural and societal challenges of adjusting is an innovative, community based grassroots program that was created in response to the lack of specific services with very limited resources or community contacts. Nah We Yone is an organization that was created to rebuild the shattered lives of African war and trauma survivors fleeing the Civil War in Sierra Leone. Using culturally informed practices, they provide psychological and support services aimed at easing the difficult transition. (Akinsulure-Smith, Smith, & Rogers, 2004, p. 119).

No doubt there are great needs all over the world for this kind of function as we daily see more and more disaster.

Unfortunately, not all perpetrators have acknowledged their traumatization. Several years ago, when I visited South Africa with a group of trauma specialists, we were aghast to find reports of former South African policemen who had moved out of the country after Nelson Mandella took over. The former policemen had, apparently, kept scrapbooks called "kill books," which were their proud collections of the many innocent victims they had tortured and killed when in power in South Africa. Sadly, humanity is not sufficiently evolved at this time to eliminate this kind of mentality. The best that we can do is to try to prevent its spread and to develop skills to provide some recovery for its victims.

AGING VICTIMS OF MASS TRAUMA

As a young woman, I lived in New York City in the time before air conditioning was easily available, and people kept their windows open on hot summer nights. I shall never forget being regularly awakened by harrowing screams coming from an apartment near mine. Disturbed by these sounds, I discussed the experience with a neighbor who was a psychiatrist. He explained to me that this woman had been in a concentration camp during the war and that those horrors would probably remain with her forever. This was my first experience of the consequences of mass trauma, but not my last, and those sounds still reverberate in my mind. During the day, the woman never talked about her experiences nor did she make any reference to her nightmares, but at night, the horrors resurfaced.

We cannot assume that time alone will heal the quality of nightmares like genocide. In fact, as you will see, the potential for the impact to worsen, or to be more visible with age, is one we must recognize. While researchers have found that older adults in the general population are a good resource during trauma situations (Norris et al., 2001), this is not necessarily the reality of older persons who have experienced severe mass trauma. These victims are a dramatic exception.

New information gives us an interesting background to measure the intense impact of an experience such as the Holocaust. For example, research done in Sydney, Australia, compares the functioning of survivors of the Holocaust, other refugees, and Australian/English-born persons of the same age. Joffe, Brodaty, Luscombe, and Ehrlich (2003) reported that on all psychological measures assessed, Holocaust survivors were functioning worse than the three groups, despite similarities in social and instrumental functioning. The more severe the trauma, the greater the level of psychological morbidity. They concluded that "despite normal social and daily functioning, psychological morbidity following massive trauma endures."

Amir and Lev-Wiesel also studied adult Holocaust victims and found that "it seems that both child survivors and adult survivors [of the Holocaust] have psychological sequelae from the extreme stress encountered in earlier stages of life" (2001). They quote Moscovitz and Krell (1990), who reported that "the memories of child survivors are often filled with painful scenes of being separated from their parents, being orphaned, being abandoned, feeling cold, starving, experiencing violence and being physically unable to move for long periods of time" (Krell, 1992). The Holocaust experience for a child might be a lifelong narrative. As the child survivors enter retirement age, some do not live as full a life as their counterparts who were not exposed to the same atrocities some 55 years ago. This was reflected in findings of more posttraumatic symptoms and higher scores regarding depression, anxiety, somatization, and anger/hostility. The present findings support earlier findings that being a child survivor is indeed a vulnerable position in late adulthood. Robinson, Rapaport-Bar-Sever, and Rapaport (1994) studied 103 child survivors about 50 years after the war and found that "most survivors still suffer from psychological distress symptoms and that their suffering is even more severe at the present time than it was immediately after the war."

Workers in homes for the aged have also been experiencing a new kind of Holocaust fallout and reawakening. Journalist Jan Wong, writing in the

Toronto Globe and Mail reports that "more than 30,000 Canadians have Alzheimer's disease or related dementia. At . . . homes for the aged which have large populations of Holocaust survivors, the loss of short-term memory condemns them once again to the death camps" (Wong, 2002). Wong quotes Dr. Michael Gordon, a gerontologist, who tells us, "For those that don't have a present any more, their past is their present." He goes on to say, "In the last ten years we are more and more involved with patients for whom the Holocaust has resurged in their consciousness. The most dramatic are those who managed to compartmentalize the experience. As they develop Alzheimer's or dementia, the Holocaust absolutely dominates their lives." Wong adds "The nursing home, aware of this phenomenon, has no gas in its dental clinic, and no one lines up for flu shots" (Wong, 2002).

This reexperiencing can create an important obstacle to help seeking in any situation. For example, in 1997, in the midst of a severely cold winter, the Province of Quebec was hit with a disastrous ice storm that wiped out electricity in almost all areas for several weeks. During that time, police and other helpers went door to door to ask aging people to come to shelters that had been set up to keep them warm and to protect them. Over and over again, they were met with the phenomenon of rejection by aging holocaust survivors, who feared that they would once again be losing their base of security in a terrifying situation over which they had no control. Memories of having been put out of their homes and taken to concentration camps prevented them from seeking a protective place. The presence of police being the messengers, even when accompanied by social workers and other helpers, aggravated this experience even more. This cohort may have to be seen as a special group and awareness of their background is important in dealing with them.

A colleague of mine, J. G., is a rape victim. She describes her reaction to her own trauma (rape):

> I grew up in a Holocaust dominated community.
>   Though my own parents were not Holocaust survivors, the members of their synagogue, many of our family friends and the parents of almost all of my friends were. Despite the terrible atrocities they experienced and witnessed, and despite the multiple effects of the traumas that undoubtedly remained, they moved forward with their lives, marrying, having children and becoming productive, if pained members of a new country and different society. These were my models after I was attacked. If they could recover to the extent they did, I could expect no less from myself. I think the models we have for coping with trauma are part of what affects the recovery process and determines to what extent we believe recovery is possible (Personal communication, 2004).

TREATING AGING GENOCIDE SURVIVORS

Pearlman, whose work in Rwanda has been cited previously, tells us that:

> Genocide is one of the most difficult human experiences to comprehend because of the malevolence that fuels it and the enormity of its consequences. It is inevitable that as we hear testimony about horrendous actions, people will again ask questions such as, Why did this happen?" "How could anyone do things like this?" "How can the world make sense if things like this can happen?" and "How do we keep this from happening again?" (2002).

In order for us to be able to take a small step toward changing the kind of the kind of mentality that can produce mass trauma, we need to be able to heal the wounds of the traumatized. Barring this, we will have to deal with an ongoing spiral of continuing pain. In chapter 7, I will go into greater detail about methods and approaches in treatment for this population as well as for other trauma-stricken populations.

LONG-TERM IMPACT OF MASS TRAUMA

Having explored mass trauma in various parts of the world, let us end this section with the words of Judith Lewis Herman:

> The ordinary human response to atrocities is to banish them from consciousness. Certain violations of the social compact are too terrible to utter aloud; this is the meaning of the word unspeakable.

> Atrocities, however, refuse to be buried. As powerful as the desire to deny atrocities is the conviction that denial does not work. Our folk wisdom and classic literature are filled with ghosts who refuse to rest in their graves until their stories are told, ghosts who appear in dreams or visions, bidding their children, "Remember me." Remembering and telling the truth about terrible events are essential tasks for both the healing of individual victims, perpetrators, and families and the restoration of the social order.

> The conflict between the will to deny horrible events and the will to proclaim them aloud is the central dialectic of psychological trauma (Herman, 1995).

TSUNAMI!

As I write this book, yet another horrendous mass trauma emerges. This time, a natural disaster threatens to break all previous records for destruction and disruption of human life.

Over the Christmas weekend in 2004, a time when one hopes that the most disastrous experiences will be airline delays (and there were many during that weekend!), a disturbing news announcement was made. The media informed us that an underwater earthquake had erupted under the Indian Ocean. Further information was that the earthquake was measured as having been a value of a nine points on the Richter Scale—one of the most powerful ever experienced.

Shortly thereafter, we started to hear of its after effects. Apparently, the earthquake caused the ocean around it to initially be pulled far away from the shores, only to return with a vengeance, drowning everything in its path, taking with it bodies, buildings, trees, and anything else that was in its way as it invaded land deep into the surrounding countries. The creation of the huge tsunami churned up the waters and turned them into menacing floods in all of the areas at hand. These included Thailand, India, Sri Lanka, Sudan, Sumatra, and other countries—14 in all. Later reports from survivors was that the oceans suddenly went further and further away from shore and then quite suddenly returned with a vengeance, going well beyond the shorelines and covering large parts of many countries.

As the day passed and more information was available, we heard horrendous things: thousands of people had drowned. One third of the people killed were children, unable to save themselves from the powerful invasion of violent, massive, churned-up waves as the oceans covered the lands. We saw violent pictures of huge waves of water viciously attacking land normally used by humans. The waters seemed relentless.

What started out as a special treat ended in death for nearly all of the passengers of the Queen of the Sea, a special railroad train that drove along the water's edge in Sri Lanka. The train was stopped by the high waters, and people climbed to the top, only to have the train overturned by the water's fury, taking the lives of all but one, a little boy. Please take a moment to imagine yourself as that little boy and experience the range of emotions that he experienced at that time and that he will live with forever. Everywhere, people reported that a 30-foot wall of water rode down on them like an "angry monster." In Sri Lanka, Indonesia, India, Thailand, Sudan, Sumatra, and myriad smaller islands, the water's fury rushed on, carrying with it thousands of drowned bodies.

In this warm climate, bodies rapidly decomposed, and mass graves were dug. The sight of human bodies being dumped into these graves by front-loader plows, like so much of yesterday's garbage, was nightmarish. Because of the fear of disease, in some places the bodies were buried before they could even be identified, leaving more thousands in severe shock, trauma, disbelief, and loss at never having any confirmation of death or the possibility of proper closure to their grief. In some areas of Indonesia alone, one-half of the residents perished. Other areas were left with not a single building standing. With bodies everywhere, survivors were often too traumatized to talk. The sight of a little girl carrying a sign seeking her missing parents and siblings was painful and almost commonplace in this horrible landscape.

A woman walked with bandages on her hands. When asked their source, she responded by saying that they were not from the tsunami itself but from having her husband's coffin pulled away from a pair of hands that wanted to hang onto him forever. It was reported that this was the biggest natural disaster of this generation.

People from North America were interviewed as they determinedly announced that they would go half way around the world to find their loved ones—but the possibility of fulfilling that dream is slight.

Some who escaped have described the disaster as apocalyptic. Days after the disaster struck, people were still dazed, depressed, devastated, having lost so much with little hope for the future. They have not yet felt the full impact of the psychological trauma or the enormous loss: loss of their families, relatives, homes, possessions—virtually the essence of their lives.

A week after the disaster, food and help were starting to arrive in the stricken countries, but thousands of people were still unaccounted for. There is numbness, disbelief, and terror in the minds of the survivors. In Sri Lanka, 600,000 homes disappeared. The numbers of lost people kept climbing. These were the ones who were too small or too weak to hold on as the water swept over them. As Beth Nissan of CNN (2004, December 30) put it, "So much life and hope has been washed away, leaving so little for the remainders to hold onto."

Shortly afterward, Oxfam sent in water for 60,000, but this was the proverbial drop in the bucket. The top emergency relief coordinator for the United Nations said that millions of people still needed assistance. Everyone feared a second wave of death from contaminated water, disease, and lack of sanitation as bodies piled up. It was feared that in the long run, one third of the deaths would be children.

Here are some of the survivors' stories:

From India:

I witnessed the most horrible scene in my life: people running for their lives, dead bodies on the road, mothers crying. I've never seen anything like this in my life. Entire fishing villages have been wiped out, huge cars floating. The bodies of children no older than seven are lying on the beach (Anonymous, 2005).

From Colombo, Sri Lanka:

My father, my mother, our driver, and I were on our way to Kataragama, where there is a famous shrine. When we got to Payagala, next to the sea, we were stopped. My father and the driver got out of the car and went near the beach. Suddenly there was a big muddy wave coming towards us. The driver got in the car but my father didn't take the wave seriously and was caught up in it. I saw him get washed away, as the three of us inside the car got drifted towards a nearby canal. The car went circling through the current and slowly filled with water. It was hit by a couple of trees that shattered the glasses. Then it came to a stop so I got out of the car through the window. Everyone was expressionless as they searched for loved ones who were with them seconds ago. I went near the canal again and saw a man helping my father who was looking exhausted, after fighting the waves, to come to safety. I have never heard or experienced such a thing before. I will never forget the huge wave as tall as a palm tree coming right towards us (Anonymous, 2005).

Now, about a month later at the time of this writing, the presumed final number of victims have been released: Approximately 200,000 people have been lost, and at least 6,000 others are still missing!

WHO AM I?

Lost Identity of Child Trauma Victims: Are We Recreating This Phenomenon?

Each of us has a name
given us by God
and by our father and our mother.
Each of us has a name
given us by the mountains
and the walls within which we live.
Each of us has a name
given to us by our enemies
and by those we love.
Each of us has a name
given us by the seasons . . .
and by the way we die.

—Zelda

As the nightmare of the tsunami mounts, more and more people around the world were appropriately touched by the faces of little children whose families have yet to be found and which may never be. Thousands of people have called international welfare organizations offering to adopt some of these helpless little ones. While this may feel like a caring, humane response, perhaps we need to consider this information: Knowing who you are and what your name is an essential piece of our existence. Studies of child trauma survivors have taught us that when these aspects are threatened, serious psychological consequences can occur.

As I walk through the park near my office every morning, I am delighted and impressed by the population of the kiddy park. I see adults, both men and women, generally older that I was when my children were toddlers, pushing swings and guiding little ones down the slides and playing games with them.

More often than not, the facial features and the skin color of these children have little, if any, correlation with that of the adults. Many of the little ones are Asiatic, adopted from China or other far away countries. They have been chosen by well-meaning parents who are generally immersed in their lives and their careers and have, for a variety of reasons, not produced children of their own. Seeing these children always warmed my heart—that is, until I read Amir and Lev-Wiesel's article (2001).

Amir and Lev-Wiesel (2001) tell us that "knowing one's name and biological parents is considered essential to personality development and psychological well-being. This study assessed posttraumatic stress disorder (PTSD) symptoms, subjective quality of life, psychological distress and potency in a group of adults who were children during the Holocaust (child Holocaust survivors), and who did not know their true identity." They report that "C," a child Holocaust survivor from Poland, was handed by her parents to a Catholic family at the age of 6 months to be hidden from the Nazis during the World War II. She was baptized and given a new name by her foster family. Her name was again changed 5 years later by the Jewish agency that brought her to Israel. All her adult life, "C" has been searching in vain for members of her original family.

As I questioned my own right to compare Holocaust children to the children in the park, I found myself reading more of Amir and Lev-Wiesel's (2001) findings, which also tell us that "situations such as this raise questions regarding the psychological effects of not knowing one's original name and identity, family members or family history. Most mental health workers agree that when the child's basic sense of security is disrupted, the (negative psychological) impact may be long term" (p. 860).

Amir and Lev-Wiesel (2001) refer to Eric Ericson: "The concept of personal identity refers to an inner sense of wholeness and security which is achieved when there is continuity between the individual's perception of self and others' perception of him/her" (Ericson, 1968). Amir and Lev-Wiesel (2001) further inform us that "if the process of identification is arrested or sabotaged there may be long-term detrimental effects on the individual. . . . Survivors with lost identity had significantly lower physiological, psychological and social Quality of Life scores and had significantly higher level of depression, anxiety and somatization compared to those who had retained their identity." Generally, one looks for prevalence of PTSD following this kind of deprivation. This was not dramatically visible in this study. However, the authors did find that

> the outcome may be the development of a different, perhaps a more subtle, and possibly more serious pattern of symptoms that expresses itself in lowered psychological well-being and Quality of Life. . . . In addition, it is possible that the time in the life of a person at which trauma occurs may affect how PTSD is evidenced. When survivors are younger, trauma may have more pervasive effects on the personality and psychological functioning and not express itself as traditional PTSD symptom of intrusive thoughts, avoidance and hyperarousal. . . . Not knowing one's identity appears to be associated with an exaggerated focus on physical well-being in holocaust survivors, and is expressed both in an increased level of somatization and a lower physical Quality of Life (p. 866).

Amir and Lev-Wiesel (2001) conclude with the statement that "not knowing one's identity can have long lasting consequences with regard to one's well-being." These children who I see in the playground have also been taken far away from their homes and placed in foreign cultures, and one can see, having read Amir and Lev-Wiesel's (2001) article, how this study applies to them as well. Are we creating a new generation of trauma victims? Do we want to do this to the little ones who have survived the tsunami and have already been traumatized by the tsunami itself, or can we find better, more creative means of keeping them close to people who they recognize?

REFERENCES

Akinsulure-Smith, R., Smith, H., & Rogers, J. (2004). *Nah We Yone, Inc: Creating hope, support and safety out of chaos.* Presented at the 20th Annual Meeting of International Society for Traumatic Stress Studies.

Amir, M., & Levi-Weisel, R. (2001). Does everyone have a name? Psychological distress and quality of life among child holocaust survivors with lost identity. *Journal of Traumatic Stress, 14*(4), 859–869.

Bolin, R. C., & Bolton, P. S. (1989). Natural disasters. In R. Gist & L. Lubin (Eds.), *Psychological aspects of disaster.* New York: Wiley.

Byant, Harvey, Dahg, et al. (1996). *Mental health intervention for disasters, National Center for PTSD Fact Sheet.*

Chopra, D. (2002). *The deeper wound.* New York: Harmony Books.

Ericson, E. (1968). *Identity, youth and crisis.* New York: Norton.

Figley, C. R. (1983). *Stress and the family. Vol. 2: Coping with catastrophe.* New York: Brunner/Mazel.

Herman, H., & Lewis, J. (1992). *Trauma and recovery.* New York: Basic Books.

Herman, J.L. (1995). Crime and memory. *Bulletin of American Academy of Psychiatry and Law,* (23)1, 5–17.

Joffe, C., Brodaty, H., Luscombe, G., & Ehrlich, F. (2003). The Sydney Holocaust study: Post-traumatic stress disorder and other psychosocial morbidity in an aged community sample. *Journal of Traumatic Stress, 16*(1), 39–47.

Krell, R. (1992). Child survivors of the holocaust: Strategies of adaptation. *Canadian Journal of Psychiatry, 38,* 384–389.

Levine, A. G.(1982). *Love canal, science, politics and people.* Toronto, Canada: D.C. Heath.

Moscowitz, S. (1995). Crime and memory. *Bulletin of American Academy of Psychiatry and Law, 23*(1).

Moscovitz, S., & Krell, R. (1990). Child survivors of the Holocaust: Psychological adaptations to survival. *Israel Journal of Psychiatry and Related Sciences, 27,* 81–91.

Norris, F. H., Byrne, C. M., Diaz, E., & Kaniasty, K. (2001). *Possible obstacles to help-seeking after trauma.* Publication of the National Center for Post-Traumatic Stress Disorder.

Pearlman, L. A., & Staub, E. (2002) *Creating paths to healing.* South Windsor, CT: Trauma Research, Education and Training Institute

Robinson, S., Rapaport-Bar-Sever, M., & Rapaport, J. (1994). The present state of people who survived the Holocaust as children. *Scandinavia, Acta Psychiatr, 89,* 242–245.

Shalev, A. Y., Tuval-Mashiach, R., & Hadar, H. (2004). Center for Traumatic Stress, Kiryat Hadassah, Israel, *Clinical Psychiatry, 65*(Suppl. 1), 4–10.

Staub, E. (1998). Breaking the cycle of genocidal violence: Healing and reconciliation. In J. Harvey (Ed.), *Perspectives on loss: A source book.* Washington, DC: Taylor & Francis.

Tiemessen, A. (2004, Fall). After Arusha, gacaca justice in post-genocide Rwanda. *African Studies Quarterly, 8*(1), 1.

Wong, J. (2002, September 28). The return of the Auschwitz nightmare. *Toronto Globe and Mail,* p. 1. Toronto, Canada.

BAKER COLLEGE OF
CLINTON TWP. LIBRARY

CHAPTER 4

Women and Trauma

War, torture, violence, poverty, diseases, discrimination and domestic abuse: these great human ills sicken the individual psyche. . . . The pathogenic power of trauma is an emerging woman's issue at the level of international policy.

—Kofi Annan (2004)

WHY "WOMEN AND TRAUMA?"

A true history of women and trauma would have to go back to the witch trials in the early days of this country, and undoubtedly to Biblical times. But suffice it to say that contemporary history is painful enough, and we will focus on that.

In chapter 1, I made reference to the universal issues of women and trauma. It was not, however until the Women's Movement of the 60s and 70s that women were encouraged to join together, and speak out about their traumatic experiences by creating consciousness-raising groups. These groups allowed many of the horrors of the reality of women's lives to surface.

Gradually, research was initiated about women's needs, allowing them to become recognized. In so doing, many of the secrets of their own sexual traumas were finally revealed and validated. Our colleague and friend, Dr. Lenore Walker, wrote poignantly about the Battered Woman Syndrome and shelters for women who were abused by their spouses were created.

Although many of these changes have been acknowledged since that time, today, at the start of 2005, women in North America and elsewhere remain uniquely at risk for traumatic experiences. Most recent information shows that, with all of our attempts at improving the situation, the National Comorbidity Survey (reported on the American Psychological Association's [APA's] Web site) indicates that the prevalence of PTSD in women is twice that of men. Women who are victims of crime and torture and concentration camp survivors suffer the highest rates of this disorder.

In addition to the potential trauma that lurks in mass violence and natural disasters and terrorist attacks, and despite the existence of women's shelters, women continue to be particularly vulnerable to specific traumas. These are created in what should be the sanctity of their homes, as well as on the streets and, most poignantly, within the military. The National Violence Against Women Study (Tjaden & Thoennes, 2000), sponsored by the National Institute of Justice and the Centers for Disease Control and Prevention, indicated that approximately 1.5 million women female partners are physically assaulted or raped by intimate partners in the United States annually. Women who are physically assaulted by an intimate partner experience an average of 3.4 separate assaults per year, and those who are raped experience 1.6 rapes annually on average (Basile, Arias, Dedsai, & Thompson, 2004).

The APA's publication *Facts About Women and Trauma* (2004) reports that "research indicates that women are twice as likely to develop PTSD, to experience a longer duration of posttraumatic symptoms, and to display more sensitivity to stimuli that remind them of trauma . . . [but] many often wait years to receive help while others never receive treatment."

Yale University's Professor H.G. Prigerson (2004) gives us further information:

> Although men experience more potentially traumatic events in their lifetime, women report more frequent and intense psychological and physical health problems following traumatic events than do men. To improve the public health of women and their children, information is needed to enhance our understanding of the ways in which exposure to trauma influences the health and functioning of women.

Quina and Brown (2005) reported at a recent International Society for Traumatic Stress Studies meeting that "community-based studies illuminate the impact of gender on the experience of trauma. Findings are that traumas experienced by women are more likely to include betrayals by someone else, and recovery is made more difficult by others' reactions of blame, stigma and disbelief." They also reported that, when disclosing a

stigmatizing experience such as rape, women often encounter negative reactions that are destructive to their healing and self-image, thus creating a
second victimization experience for the victim. In chapter 6, we discuss the
structure and value of social support in dealing with crisis and trauma; this
information is significant in its role of further undermining an already injured woman.

The impact of childhood trauma has been found to be of greater significance in women than men. A recent study by Hobfoil, Schumm, and
Stiners (2004) demonstrated that "childhood trauma undermines psychosocial resources in adulthood. . . ." Women whose resources are under-
mined are, in turn "more vulnerable to both major stressors in adulthood
and traumatic stressors. . . . When major stress or traumatic stress occurs in
women's lives, those who had childhood traumatic experiences lack resources to combat the deleterious impact of the new challenges" (p. 115).

When I visited South Africa several years ago, domestic rape was quite
prevalent and almost taken for granted. One group of women told us that
after being raped, their only source of healing was to meet with other
women in church and to pray together. Another group was amazed to hear
that in North America, men could be sent to jail for raping. What amazed
them most was that these men could be imprisoned for raping their own
spouses. This may make us feel smug and superior, perhaps even safer, but
the reality of women's experience, even in the most sophisticated nations of
the world, is that women are victimized and traumatized much more often
than we can imagine.

At a recent meeting of the International Society for Traumatic Stress
Studies, Dr. Mary Armsworth (2004) quite directly described the condition
of many women in the world today: "The pathogenic power of trauma is an
emerging women's issue at the level of international policy. . . . Many of the
state members of the United Nations today are not democracies and still
embrace the chattel status of women, meaning 'movable property' of men.
This dehumanized status is the root cause of enormous trauma to the
world's women."

Violence against women is universal, and no country, no matter how
proud they may be of their sense of equality or liberation, is free of these
behaviors.

Tompson and colleagues (2004) recently reported that "consistent with
previous research, women with PTSD self-reported a greater number of interpersonal violent acts than women without PTSD. The male spouses of
women with PTSD reported (and the women with PTSD corroborated)

higher levels of interpersonal violence than male partners of women without PTSD." So the violence and abuse goes on and on, in what appears to be a self-perpetuating manner.

STATISTICS, WOMEN, AND TRAUMA

One of my colleagues, Dr. Ken Pope, has provided the following material (originally created by Amnesty International), which can help us to grasp the realities of violence against women. If we can imagine a scaled down world as a global village of 1,000 people,

- 500 would be women. (It would be 510, but 10 were never born due to gender selective abortion or died in infancy due to neglect.)
- 167 would be beaten or in some way exposed to violence in their lifetime.
- 199 of the women would be victims of rape or attempted rape in their lifetime.

Dr. Pope provides us with this additional data:

- up to 70% of female murder victims are killed by their male partners
- every 90 seconds in the United States a women is raped
- During wartime, 80% of the refugees are women and children
- More than 135 million girls and women have undergone female genital mutilation and an additional 2 million girls and women are at risk each year (Courtesy of Dr. Ken Pope, Personal communication).

It is also known that in the United States, 16% of women report rapes to the police. Of those who do not, nearly 50% would do so if they could be assured that their names and private details would not be released publicly. In the United Kingdom, 13% of all raped women report the assault to the police. Seventy-nine countries have no (or unknown) legislation against domestic violence. Marital rape is recognized specifically as a crime in only 51 countries.

Relative to men, women are more likely to be injured if they are victimized by an intimate partner than if they are assaulted by a non-intimate (Saltzman, 1995) and are 13 times more likely to suffer an injury from an intimate partner than from an accident (Stark, Flitcraft, & Frazier, 1979). Injuries from intimate partner victimization can include bruises, scratches, burns, broken bones, miscarriages and knife and gunshot wounds (Crowell & Burgess, 1996).

THE WOMEN AND TRAUMA PROJECT

Residence XII is one of many organizations affiliated with the Women and Trauma Project. Here is how the organization's mission is described:

> As many as 80% of women seeking treatment for drug abuse have experienced either sexual or physical assault. These experiences often lead to nightmares, an inability to stop thinking about the event, feeling numb, being easily frightened and jumpy, or feeling depressed, worried, or hopeless. These are just a few signs of . . . posttraumatic stress disorder.
>
> Residence XII has been selected as the only site west of the Mississippi to be a part of the Women and Trauma Project, an important study through the National Drug Abuse Treatment Clinical Trails Network. The National Institute on Drug Abuse (NIDA) Women and Trauma Project is exciting because it looks specifically at the treatment of women with substance abuse and PTSD.
>
> The empowerment of women has always been a central value to Residence XII, a cornerstone of bringing gender-specific treatment to our clients and developing a program that can best serve women. We have embraced the NIDA Women and Trauma Project as a way to empower women and women's treatment through research.
>
> Historically, most scientific research has studied primarily white, middle class men. As a result, the treatments emerging from those research projects do not always address and respond to the needs of women. The nationwide Women and Trauma Project will compare two different interventions designed specifically for women: "Seeking Safety" and "Women's Health Education." Residence XII will provide these interventions in addition to our usual treatment. We, along with NIDA, are working to see how well the interventions help women reduce their substance use, stress, and other emotional problems as well as increase their treatment attendance. About 480 women will be enrolled in the project at several sites nationwide, including about 60 volunteers from Residence XII (Valente, 2004).

This is indeed a worthwhile project. There are many more pieces of data such as we have demonstrated, but I think that this material suffices to set the scene for the material we are about to present.

TRAUMA AND WOMEN'S HEALTH

Kimerling and Baumrind (2004) report that "Research is only beginning to elucidate the relationship between PTSD and women's health status." They recently presented research on associations of PTSD with common indicators of women's health status in a diverse community sample of women. They explored potentially unique effects for intimate partner violence and sexual abuse/assault.

The 3,800 California women, aged 18 to 44, participated in a survey that included exploration of childhood sexual and physical abuse, sexual assault, physical assault, and detailed information regarding partner violence in the past year. They found that PTSD was related to health status indicators when adjusted for the effects of ethnicity, marital status, education, and poverty. PTSD was significantly associated with fair or poor health status, failure to receive a routine health checkup in the past year, smoking, and problem drinking beyond the healthy range. They concluded that PTSD is associated with poor health, access to health care, and health risk behaviors.

An article by Green et al. (1998) reports research on 160 women with both early stage breast cancer and a history of trauma. Given a battery of psychological tests, the researchers found that these women demonstrated psychiatric problems that arose while experiencing early stage breast cancer. The psychiatric problems were linked to their traumatic experiences. When one realizes that both cancer and traumatic experiences are potentially life threatening, this finding should come as no surprise.

Another recent study from Taft (2004) found a significant association between physical assault, psychological aggression, and higher levels of PTSD symptoms among battered women as well as a strong correlation between severe health injuries and physical assault. Psychological aggressions were also related to poor physical health.

Casey and Resick (2004), as well as others, have recently presented information reinforcing the clinical impressions many of us who work with women have observed: "Considerable evidence indicates that women who experience relationship abuse are at risk for poor physical health," and "PTSD symptoms play an important role with respect to the development of physical health symptoms."

WOMEN, TRAUMA, AND THE MILITARY

In response to a growing awareness of sexual assault in the military, Congress included in the Veterans Health Care Act of 1992 the authority and priority for providing counseling and treatment for sexual trauma.

Specifically, the law states that the secretary of the Department of Veterans Affairs should provide sexual trauma treatment to "overcome psychological trauma, which in the judgment of a mental health professional employed by the department, resulted from a physical assault of a sexual nature, battery of a sexual nature, or sexual harassment which occurred while the veteran was serving on active duty."

Despite this fact, Fontana and Rosenhek (1998) found that

The stressful experiences of women serving in the military have been a focus of increasing concern. A model of the impact of stress related to the military duty and stress related to sexual abuse and harassment on the development of PTSD among female veterans was evaluated. A total of 63% reported experiences of physical sexual harassment during military service, 43% reported rape or attempted rape. Both duty-related and sexual stress were found to contribute separately and significantly to the development of PTSD. *Sexual stress was found to be almost four times as influential in the development of PTSD as duty related stress.*

Some journalists have reported that women in the military were often raped, and many of those who were assaulted eventually left the services. Their attackers, however, remained, and often went on to be promoted.

Dr. Sharon Wills (2004) recently presented material that dealt with the emerging issues of the continuing traumatic experiences of women in the military. She tells us the following:

In the past few years the once-taboo subject of sexual violence perpetrated against women in the military has received increased public attention. Through the Veterans' Millennium Healthcare Bill, Congress mandated that the Veterans Administration screen and offer treatment to all military veterans reporting sexual abuse. To date more than 34,000 women have screened positive for Military-Related Sexual Trauma (MST). Recent Senate hearings have increased awareness of MST in women serving on active duty, and in the first 18 months of armed conflict in Iraq, Afghanistan and Kuwait roughly 112 rapes were reported which likely under-represents the actual number of rapes occurring. This evidence has strong implications for systemic policy changes in the military and VA if they are to more effectively prevent, respond to and treat survivors of military-related sexual violence.

HOMELESSNESS

Not surprisingly, homelessness, particularly in women, is often accompanied by violence and has been shown to be related to PTSD.

Research suggests that women who are homeless may be exposed to higher rates of violence and therefore may have higher rates of PTSD than other women. A study by Jackson et al. (2003) examines the rates of PTSD (as measured by Foa's Posttraumatic Diagnostic Scale) and their correlates in a unique sample of homeless women, primarily African American, who have children.

When interviewed, 25% acknowledged needing trauma-related services in the past 3 months, but only half of these women received such services. Half of the women in this sample reported symptoms suggestive of a PTSD diagnosis. Seventy-five percent of the sample experienced physical violence from a family member or familiar person; 60% of these women said this trauma first occurred before the age of 18. More than half of the sample (58%) reported sexual abuse by someone known to them, and 85% experienced this before the age of 18 (Jackson et al., 2003).

The Women of the Omarska Camp

"When I got home I smelled of death—even my dog ran away from me." This is how a Muslim woman who was imprisoned in the Omarska Prison Camp during the Bosnia-Herzegovina horrors describes herself in the 1997 documentary, *Calling the Ghost*. These women, imprisoned in the Serbian camp Omarska, were rounded up and taken there simply because of their ethnic background. Once there, they were herded into rooms, tortured, forced to watch the torture of their cohorts and repeatedly raped by the commander of the camp. Each night the commander would enter their room and each would be terrified to see which one he would choose for that night. Once he made the choice and took her out she was not only raped by him but by all of his underlings throughout the night. This was a part of the "Ethnic cleansing" that was ongoing at that time. They reported that they came out of the camps completely different women, injured in body and soul, living in fear of anyone walking behind them. Many felt so ashamed by the experience that they became silent, unable to speak (Link TV, 1997).

Although many raped women remained silent, some in this group were true Phoenixes (see chapter 6). Gradually, they came together and felt the need to tell their story, which was both healing and empowering. Eventually, they took their case to the International War Crimes Tribunal at the Hague. Although the Tribunal was not effective, the empowering experience allowed them to carry on with their lives, and to tell their stories.

THE TRAUMA OF FORCED MIGRATION AND WAR

As we have seen in previous sections, forced migration can have a severely traumatic impact.

Dr. Judith Pilowsky is a Toronto-based psychologist who is originally from Chile and who specializes in working with immigrants, refugees, and victims of violence and torture. She tells us

> when the political and social become personal, the impact of social and political trauma is transformed to physical difficulty and emotional conflicts. There are devastating consequences to leaving one's country against one's will—the world is no longer a safe place for women who have had this experience. Women lose family and social support; they are not there when elderly parents get sick or die; their children grow up without grandparents.
>
> These losses are often compounded by the barriers to finding treatment and support in their new country. There are not a lot of multicultural and ethnically diverse services, and those that exist are expensive or have long waiting lists. These conditions make women vulnerable to physical and psychological difficulties (2002).

This is just an example of the impact of forced migration. When we consider the multiple areas of the world that are either currently or recently under siege and the vulnerability of women's lives, the enormity of the need to develop effective methods of healing becomes apparent. If we could educate the world about the horrors of trauma and have them altered, that would be ideal.

Some years ago, I had the privilege of being the president of the Women's Center of Montreal. In that capacity, I had a direct connection with the faces, hearts, and minds of women refugees. The sense of terror behind their eyes, their fear for their own ability to survive and protect their children, and the sense of helplessness in trying to assimilate into a culture with totally foreign languages still stay with me.

Professor Maria Olujic of the University of Zagreb in Croatia has written a moving article titled "Women, Rape and War: The Continued Trauma of Refugees and Displaced Persons" (1993). In it, she says

> rape has been used as a tactic of terror in many wars. . . . Rape was a weapon of terror as the German Hun marched through Belgium in World War I; gang rape was part of the orchestrated riots of Kristallnacht which marked the beginning of Nazi campaigns against Jews. It was a weapon of revenge as the Russian Army marched to Berlin in World War II, [and] when the Japanese raped Chinese women in the city of Nanking, when the Pakistani Army battled Bangladesh, and when the American GI's made rape in Vietnam a "standard operating procedure" aimed at terrorizing the population into submission" (Bergman 1974, p. 69). But in these wars rape did not receive the widespread publicity it has in the ongoing war in the former Yugoslavia. Rape is not only important on

individual, familial, community levels but also the international level, because all sides in the conflict use the stories of rape as propaganda for political gain. In addition, governments need to make policy in response to rapes, regulate treatment of victimized women, access to abortion or adoption, and legal responses to the aggressors. Furthermore war rapes and gender-based violence need to be defined as a form of torture and a war crime.

It is over a decade since Madame Olujic wrote these stirring words, and not much has changed in women's lives in respect to protecting themselves and their sisters around the world from the horrors of rape. I write these words in the hope that some reader, considerably younger than myself, will take up the challenge and help to eradicate this aspect of horror in women's lives. As Judith Lewis Herman (1992) has taught us, "Traumatic reactions occur when taking action is senseless. If it is neither possible to put up resistance nor to flee, the self-defence mechanism of a human being is over-taxed and breaks down in a state of chaos."

DIVERSITY

Angela Robertson is the executive director of Sistering, an organization that provides a wide range of support services to homeless, under-housed and low-income women. Here are some of her thoughts on women of diversity:

> Often only certain women are seen as diverse women, which influences the services created. Sometimes we only identify women of color and don't begin to talk about the intersectionality of who we are and what constitutes our diversity. There are many other, less obvious circumstances that marginalize women—poverty, sexual orientation, immigration status, religion, language, or working in unsafe conditions. Even women's homelessness can be invisible, such as when we sleep on a series of friends' couches. All of these circumstances can be sources of ongoing trauma (Personal communication, 2004).

A generic one-size-fits-all approach will not address all of these different needs. "Many women who have experienced violence and abuse live in ongoing disempowerment," Robertson says, "because of so many other factors—racism, poverty, mental illness, sexual orientation. A generic structure is not set up with their interests in mind."

These concepts are important for us to keep in mind, particularly as we hear discussion of diverse women who are traumatized or when we interact with these women in our personal or professional lives.

PEACEKEEPERS?

As I came to the end of this chapter, I discovered yet another horrendous violation of women, again perpetrated by those we assume would be protectors. An article by Marc Lacey in *The New York Times* reports that United Nations peacekeepers assigned to the Congo have been raping innocent young girls and women. He reports the following: "In the corner of the tent where she says a soldier forced himself on her, Helen, a frail fifth-grader with big eyes and skinny legs remembers seeing a blue helmet. . . . The UN peacekeeper who tore off her clothes had used a cup of milk to lure her . . . It was her favorite drink but one her family could rarely afford" (December, 2004).

Lacey further reports that apparently the United Nations had reported 150 allegations of sexual abuse perpetrated by United Nations peacekeepers in a rather short period of time. Lacey also notes that "the raping of women and girls is an all too common tactic in the war raging in the Congo's jungles, involving numerous militia groups. In Bunia, a program run by UNICEF has treated 2,000 victims of sexual violence in recent months. But it is not just the militia members who have been preying on the women. So, too, local women say, have been some of the soldiers brought in to keep the peace."

Who, then, are the "good guys"?

REFERENCES

Annan, K. (2004). War, peace, prevention, practice and policy. Human Dignity and Humanitarian Studies: Trauma Intervention in War and Peace.

Armsworth, M. (2004, November). *Women and trauma: Domestic, international and military policy.* 20th Annual Symposium of the International Society for Traumatic Stress Studies, New Orleans, LA.

Basile, K. C., Arias, I., Dedsai, S., & Thompson, M. P. (2004, October). The differential association of intimate partner physical, sexual, psychological and stalking violence and posttraumatic stress symptoms in a nationally representative sample of women. *Journal of Traumatic Stress, 17*(5), 413–423.

Bergman, G. (1974). In M. B. Olujic. (1998, Spring). Women, rape, and war: The continued trauma of refugees and displaced persons in Croatia. *Anthropology of East Europe Review, 13*(1).

Bowery Productions. (1998). *Calling the ghost: The women of Omarska,* [Documentary]. M. Jacobson & K. Jelincic (Producers). Presented on LINK TV, December 2004.

Brownmiller, S. (1975). *Men, women and rape.* New York: Simon and Schuster.

Casey, T., & Resick, P. (2004, November). *PTSD and physical health among help-*

seeking battered women. 20th Annual Symposium of the International Society for Traumatic Stress Studies, New Orleans, LA.

Crowell, N., & Burgess, A. (Eds.). (1996). *Understanding violence against women.* National Research Council, Washington, DC: National Academy Press.

Facts about women and trauma. (2004). Factsheet for the American Psychological Association.

Fontana, A., & Rosenhek, R. (1998). Duty-related and sexual stress in the etiology of PTSD among women veterans who seek treatment. *Psychiatric Services, 49,* 658–662. Quoted in 20th Annual Symposium of the International Society for Traumatic Stress Studies, New Orleans, LA.

Green, B. L., Krupnick, J. L., Rowland, J. H., Epstein, S. A., Stockton, P., Spertus, I., et al. (1998). *Trauma history as a predictor of psychologic symptoms in women.* Washington, DC: Department of Psychiatry, Georgetown University.

Herman, J. L. (1992). *Trauma and recovery.* New York: Basic Books.

Hobfoil, S., Schumm, J., & Stiners, L. P. (2004, November). *Childhood trauma, resource loss and adult vulnerability among women.* National Center for PTSD, Dartmouth Medical School, Interpersonal Violence and Women's Health, presented to the 20th Annual Meeting of the International Society for Traumatic Stress Studies, New Orleans, LA.

Jackson, E., Crowder, C., Sleath, B. L., Galloway, J. H., Thomans, K. C., et al. (2003, November). *Trauma history, PTSD, and access to mental health services in homeless women with children.* 131st Annual Meeting, American Psychological Association.

Kimerling, R., & Baumring, K. (2004). *PTSD and women's health indicators.* 20th Annual Meeting of the International Society for Traumatic Stress Studies, New Orleans, LA.

Lacey, M. (2004). A shameful thing for the UN. *The New York Times,* reprinted in the *Montreal Gazette,* December 19, 2004.

Lichtenthal, W. G., Cruess, D. G., & Prigerson, H. G. (2004). Summary of Traumatic Stress Literature, in Australian Center of Posttraumatic Mental Health.

National Comorbidity Survey. (2004). Washington, DC: American Psychological Association.

Olujic, M. B. (1993). Women, rape and war, the continued trauma of refugees and displaced persons in Croatia. *Anthropology of East Europe Review, 13*(1).

Pilowsky, J. (2002, March 7). *The trauma of forced migration.* Paper presented at Women and Trauma: Challenging Boundaries, Healing Wounds, Taking Action. Centre for Addiction and Mental Health.

Quina, K., & Brown, L. (2005, November). *The impact of gender on trauma and recovery experiences.* 20th Annual Meeting of the International Society for Traumatic Stress Studies, New Orleans, LA.

Robertson, A. (2001). Sistering, Toronto-Peel Mental Health Implemenation Task Force. Retrieved from www.sistering.org.

Saltzman, L. E. (1995). Costs of intimate partner violence in the United States. *JAMA*, 3043, 3045.

Stark, E., Flitcraft, A. H. & Frazier, W. (1979). Medicine and patriarchal violence: The social construction of a "private" event. *International Journal of Health Sciences, 9*, 461–493.

Taft, C., Resick, P., Mechanic, M., Vogt, D., & Schnurr, P. (2004, November). *PTSD and physical health among among help seeking battered women*. Paper presented at 20th Annual Meeting of the International Society for Traumatic Stress Studies, New Orleans, LA.

Tjaden, P., & Thoennes, N. (2004). *Stalking in America: Findings from the National Violence Against Women Survey,* 1998. Presented at the International Society for Traumatic Stress Studies, 20th Annual Meeting, New Orleans, LA, November 14–18, 2004.

Tompson, W., Feldman, M., Malesky, L., Beckham, J., et al. (2004). *Interpersonal violence in women with and without PTSD*. Symposium presented at 20th Annual Meeting of the International Society for Traumatic Stress Studies, New Orleans, LA.

Valente, A. (2004). The Women and Trauma Project at Residence XII, *Summer Newsletter.*

Walker, L. (1979). *The battered woman syndrome*. New York: Springer Publishing.

Wills, S. (2004, November). *Women and war: The high cost of sexual violence in the military.* Paper presented at 20th Annual Meeting of the International Society for Traumatic Stress Studies, New Orleans, LA.

CHAPTER 5

Life-Threatening Illness: Cancer and the Trauma From Within

First, you cry.

—Betty Rollin (1976)

IMPACT AND ROLE CHANGE OF THE THERAPIST

When you get a call from a patient diagnosed with cancer or from a family member, a loved one, or a good friend asking to see you professionally, before you can even respond honestly and appropriately to that call, the first person you have to confront is yourself. Being mere mortals and, in that sense no different from cancer patients, our initial free association to the word *cancer* often is the word *death*. And you, the professional, have to drop your protective professional cloak, your well-trained understanding of "self" and "other," and go into your soul to explore your deepest feelings about cancer. You must go to that scary place within each of us, the place that says "That could be me!" You must look at it and feel it and understand it.

And after you have dealt with that place, after you have acknowledged its existence, after you have allowed yourself to fully experience the meaning and depth of the situation—to feel the quality of terror and fear that the diagnosis evokes, not only in your patient but in yourself—only then can you start to work with your cancer patients, their families, and their friends. Because that self-knowledge will change your life, it will alter you, it will

49

destroy what the author has named the "magic bubble of invisible invincibility," but it will make you come to grips with your mortality—and if you are fortunate, it will make you a more humane human being. This experience will give you access to the taste, the smell, and the feel of facing a life-threatening trauma.

CANCER AS TRAUMA

A diagnosis of cancer, of whatever kind, and at whatever stage of the life cycle, is potentially a trauma. Having a life-threatening illness such as cancer may differ from other kinds of traumatic events in that the threat is "ongoing and anchored in the present and the future, rather than in the past, and the threat arises from one's own body rather than an external source." (Green et al., 1998). The initial impact of a diagnosis of cancer means "death" "I am facing a death sentence" to many people.

Recent research by Koopman, Butler, Classen, Giese-Davis, and colleagues (2002) in an article titled "Traumatic Symptoms Among Women With Recently Diagnosed Primary Breast Cancer" indicates that the

> emotional, cognitive, and social impact of cancer may compound its medical effects and negatively affect a patient's psychosocial adjustment. . . . For some cancer patients the process associated with with being diagnosed and treated may be sufficiently traumatizing that they produce posttraumatic stress reactions such as avoidance and intrusive symptoms.

The American Psychiatric Association (APA) has acknowledged the potential for life-threatening illness such as cancer to be traumatic stressors by including these illnesses among the event exposure criteria for the diagnosis of posttraumatic stress disorder.

Populations and Treating Modalities

Facing the reality of the prevalence of cancers like breast cancer is an important step in your dealing with it as a practitioner. When I was growing up in New York, the subways had an advertisement that said "One out of every 12 women will get breast cancer." My friends and I, smug in our adolescence, would count out the women in the car and heave a sigh of relief that we would not be that "one"! Denial is a great friend, but it cannot last forever!

Today, according to governmental statistics, the occurrence of breast cancer in women is

    at age 40 . . . 1/217
    at age 50 . . . 1/50
    at age 60 . . . 1/24
    at age 70 . . . 1/14
    at age 85 . . . 1/9

The odds are frightening, and as therapists, we must become aware of them as well as learn what we need to know about dealing with them.

No matter what type of cancer is diagnosed, the people closest to the patient are suddenly thrown into the position of being secondary victims of trauma. Our work in dealing with trauma has shown us that these victims go through the same stages of traumatic response as the primary victims themselves. Both patients and loved ones will probably experience a sense of denial and undoing as their own personal "magic bubble" is shattered. No longer is cancer something that happens only to others, it has now happened to them. One reaction to this may be to shoot the messenger, with considerable feelings of conflict toward the doctor, at whom they now feel both anger and dependency. This may well be followed by a sense of mourning—a sense, quite realistic, that their lives will never again be the same.

Therapists working in this modality respond in ways that are unique and different from that of traditional therapy. Dr. Alastair Cunningham, a cancer researcher and author of *The Healing Journey* (2000), has developed three stages of self-help: getting connected, searching for meaning, and taking control.

WORKING WITH CANCER PATIENTS: PATIENTS' NEEDS AND THERAPISTS' SKILLS

In our work with cancer patients, we have developed a series of principles that we have found to be effective. These are the following:

1. urgency
2. normalization
3. focus on strength and empowerment
4. flexibility and involvement
5. emphasis on hope and expectations
6. facilitation of resources

I will explore each of these principles.

Urgency

The person with cancer feels that her or his problem-solving ability is over-whelmed and needs immediate response to feel that something is being done, that something is changed, or can be changed—that there is some movement. She or he may feel immobilized and need to emerge even from the initial contact with you with some jointly arrived at clear position on what needs to be addressed or done. This does not necessarily allow for casual history taking. When a person has been given a diagnosis of cancer, all responses are magnified. The life-threatening potential creates a very special kind of immediacy. The here-and-now is the medium.

Your work will include an action orientation that may sometimes take the form of a plan, or perhaps an exercise. It is important that the clients leave feeling that they have been heard and responded to. They need to feel that they have a partner in their race against time. Patients have reported to me that taking home a new skill, whether it be a relaxation tool, a mantra, or any other kind of intervention was regarded as helpful.

Normalization

The client is temporarily overwhelmed by a life situation that overtaxes her or his problem-solving ability. She or he is not a pathological individual who must be diagnosed and treated. The goal is not to cure a neurosis or psychosis but to facilitate the enhancement of the quality of her or his life and give a sense of control over this terrifying experience. His or her experience of this situation is entirely normal, namely, trying to make sense of an abnormal situation; being a part of that situation does not make one abnormal.

Focus on Strength and Empowerment

In all situations such as these, as therapists, we focus not on clients' weaknesses or pathologies but rather on their strengths. We help them to regain their own focus on those strengths and on their remaining stabilities, and to learn to use them to rebuild. We reinforce positives even if the only visible positives were the clients' choosing to see a therapist. At a time when all of their stabilities appear to be disintegrating, we help them to rediscover old stabilities and to create new ones, and we work with all of these.

Flexibility and Involvement

As a therapist in this type of situation, you are far more actively involved with the client then is the traditional therapist. You must do "whatever the client can not do for herself, and no more" (Parad, 1965).

Be prepared to be creative in your interventions and skill building. Do whatever is necessary for the client at that time, as well as to be a resource person for all kinds of relevant information, from the impact of nutrition to the best available surgical treatment. You must even be prepared to accompany your client for treatment if this is absolutely necessary. Even as you foster self-reliance in the patient, you must be available as a "benign person, an effective ombudsman" (Shneidman, 1985)—not only to provide the client with all kinds of information, but, if the client is unable to do so, make the connections yourself. Some very traditional therapists may be uncomfortable with this approach. This work, however, is based on the crisis intervention–trauma response model, which does not allow for traditional work in the comfort of an office when interventions may be needed elsewhere. It requires a considerable amount of flexibility and versatility.

Emphasis on Hope and Expectations

A sense of hopelessness/helplessness is a part of these situations. It is therefore important for you, the therapist, to do everything in your power to maintain a sense of hope. Hope is a crucial element in the positive outcome of any crisis or trauma, and it is essential for therapists to encourage it. Puryear (1979) says, "Promise nothing but expect a great deal." Assume that you will, together, be able to make some headway in this situation. Be realistic about your own expectations of your own progress as well as the client's. Making Headway may not necessarily prolong life, but it can certainly enhance the quality of life. However, even as you are doing this, you must stay in touch with the legitimacy of the client's distress; avoid an attitude of "there, there—it will pass," which is trivialization. Help clients reconnect with aspects of themselves that they may be overlooking because of the overwhelming presence of the traumatic situations.

Facilitation of Resources

Resources can be internal, interpersonal, informational, community-based, and spiritual.

Internal resources refer to facilitation and building of the patient's coping skills such as relaxation, visualization, self-hypnosis, problem solving, communication, and so on. These skills give the patient a sense of control in this difficult situation.

Interpersonal resources protect the client from a sense of loneliness and isolation. These feelings occur when a patient is suddenly thrust out of the "normal" population into the population of the ill.

People in crisis or trauma are particularly vulnerable and can easily be helped or hindered by responses from their immediate environment. The helper needs to understand the aspects of an effective support system in order to help patients create and use it. Thus, an often crucial piece of the client's function at this time comes from the use of a support network. In chapter 4, we defined support as "access to and experience of a relationship that is appropriate to the level of interpersonal need experienced by an individual at any given time." The three levels identified were casual, functional-social, and validation (Wainrib, 1975).

It is important for therapists to recognize that they, too, are a significant piece of that support system for the duration of the trauma. During trying periods, they may have to be available at any time, any place, and most particularly, they have to be most responsive to patients' needs.

Informational support includes helping clients to have access to information about illness, treatments, and alternative treatments, as well as other informational need that they may express.

Community support requires accessing resources such as self-help groups and information sources. Therapists may help clients to make these connections.

Spiritual support refers to encouraging the use of the client's existing belief systems. Remember that every potentially traumatic situation is also a crisis of faith. If the client has any kind of spiritual belief, encourage the use of that belief. Michael Lerner (1994), in his book, *Choices in Healing,* tells us that "cancer means facing the uncertainty of illness, the probability of pain, and the possibility of death. For many people, these encounters evoke profound shifts in consciousness that may be called spiritual." In a later chapter, I will discuss spirituality in more depth, but at this point, it is an important concept to be aware of for this modality.

In working with cancer patients, therapists must assume new roles. They need to drop some of their clinical training and use their life as a springboard to understanding the patient at this time. Let us remember the beautiful words of Martin Buber: "In human society at all its levels, persons confirm one another in a practical way, to some extent or other in their personal qualities or capacities, and a society may be termed human in the measure in which its members confirm one another. . . . Actual humanity exists only where this capacity unfolds" (Buber, 1958).

And Dr. Alastair Cunningham reminds us that "the role of the health professional, whatever his or her primary discipline . . . can be much more than mere repair. He or she can be teacher and a guide in the discovery of new meaning in illness and in life. A teacher is simply a fellow traveler with a few more years of experience than the student. If he or she is to function in this role he or she must be engaged sincerely in seeking personal meaning" (Cunningham, 2000).

SKILLS THERAPISTS NEED

Therapists must also be free to shift from psychotherapeutic skills to psychoeducational skills as they move from a traditional professional role to that of a guide and journey along with the patient. No matter what your orientation, in this kind of work, the sense of connection is primary. Working with cancer patients also means learning a great deal about treatments, about medical systems, and about alternative treatments.

Therapists must learn about professional and community resources that may be needed by the patient and learn to do their own networking with these resources. Also, therapists need to search themselves about the meaning of "meaning" and how that may cause them to look at issues of their own feelings and to be open to other interpretations.

Flexibility and creativity are at the core of the model. Therapists must understand as well, that the diagnosed patient is not their only concern, as we mentioned previously. Families, friends, and loved ones of the patient who are now secondary victims have been shown in studies to experience stages of psychological response that are very similar to the primary victim.

In my previous book, we made reference to the Van Gennep (1960) model of "mourning, confusion and reemergence." We said that

> mourning is generally considered to be an end product, not a beginning. But mourning is the first part of the necessary transition in crisis and trauma. . . . Whether the situation can create positive change or negative loss, there is always . . . mourning necessary. . . . Much as one thinks "make it yesterday" when first confronted with this situation, the reality is that yesterday will never again exist (Wainrib, in Wainrib & Bloch, 1998).

A simple but significant change in the way you will work is the location of your work. No longer will you be confined to your safe, secure womb of an office. You will be where the patient needs you to be. In 1991, when I was chairing the Gender Issues Committee of Division 42 APA, we became aware of the great need for educating psychologists about breast cancer. In the process of putting together the book, *Breast Cancer: A Psychological Treatment Manual* (Haber et al., 1993), I got calls from colleagues telling me that patients had asked them to accompany them to treatments, to visit them at home, and to perform other functions atypical of traditional therapy. They would say, "Do you call this 'therapy'?" and I would simply answer them, "No, this is Trauma Response." Mobile you must be—you may see patients in the office but also at home or in the hospital, if necessary, when they go to treatments. Sometimes this creates some role confusion with the hospital staff. One day I was visiting one of my patients who was hospitalized with breast cancer. The nurse opened the door, and said "Oh, I see you have a visitor. Perhaps she could help in washing your hair." My patient, indignant, replied, "Dr. Wainrib does not wash hair!"

You will be intervening with a variety of populations, in a variety of modalities, and at a variety of intervention points. The populations you will be working with will include patients, spouses/partners, family, children, and staff. You may see them individually or in combinations such as couples, families, and groups, at times simultaneously. You must be flexible as well in the kinds of modalities that are appropriate at different times.

You may be called upon at intervention points such as the following:

- at the diagnostic process
- during the treatment and at the end of it
- giving and getting diagnostic information
- helping to understand information needs

After the information is internalized, it may well be followed by a sense of mourning. Confusion about their futures, their choices, and perhaps even their identities may also be present. Eventually, with the help of a good professional guide who can help them to access their own internal resources, a good support system, and compassionate healers, we can hope that a new sense of self will emerge and that the sense of confusion will lead to a new stronger sense of identity for a client.

That, however, is far away from the initial experience. It is a goal for the practitioner to hold long before the patient will even be able to fantasize it.

Patients' internal reactions to the diagnosis are further complicated by whether they are successful in dealing with a very complicated medical system. Technical advances over the past 40 years have made important changes in the treatment and, in some cases, the life expectancy of people with a diagnosis of cancer. At the same time, the growing technicalization of cancer treatment has isolated the patient from important psychological functions. To quote Lewis Thomas, "To many patients stunned by the diagnosis, suffering numerous losses and discomforts, moved from place to place for one procedure after another, the experience is bewildering and frightening: at worst it is like being trapped in the workings of a giant machine" (1974).

GENDER, FAMILY SYSTEMS, AND TRAUMA

Prostate cancer is potentially life threatening. A diagnosis of any kind of cancer immediately creates the fear of death and loss in both the patient and their loved ones; a man faces death, and a woman faces severe loss and widowhood. All involved are facing a potentially traumatic situation, and they respond accordingly.

Prostate cancer is known as the silent killer, primarily because it can develop with no dramatic symptoms but also because men, by dint of their own socialization, may tend to ignore their medical problems. As one of our interviewees told us, "Symptoms are usually ignored because men are taught to keep complaints to a minimum. They are supposed to be macho, not cry or express pain." While some of us may feel that these reactions are stereotypical and out of date, we need to remember that prostate cancer generally strikes after the age of 50 and becomes more prevalent each decade after that, so that our cohort of patients are coming from a traditional masculine model.

Prostate cancer attacks the source of a man's sense of manhood just at a time in his life that he may already be having concerns about his virility (male midlife reactions). It impacts on his relationship with a partner because of the unspoken rules of the man-woman ecology. In an overwhelming majority of cases, men turn to the women in their lives for help in researching the illness, providing emotional relief, and communicating with others. This is one of the unspoken ways in which the man-woman balance has always worked. But for women, their partner's diagnosis of prostate cancer can cause their experience of the relationship system to break down. They also have to face the demands of a disease that threatens a man that they love and that threatens him in the area of his self-esteem and emotional equilibrium. At the same time, they are experiencing a mutual trauma that, regardless of its outcome, may cause an irrevocable disruption in their lives together. While men are struggling with anger, fear, depression, flight, guilt, and so on, women are struggling with emotional isolation, panic, despair, and resentment as well as the fear and, yes, the anger.

Difficulties for the couple are aggravated from the moment of diagnosis of prostate cancer. Unlike many cancers, there is no consensus amongst the medical community about treatment choices for this disease. The combination of this confusion plus the approach of informed consent presents the patient and his partner with an enormous burden. As one patient said, "When I have a broken leg, the doctor gives me the diagnosis and tells me that he will put it in a cast, but with prostate cancer, the doctor gives me the diagnosis and then tells me that I have to make my own decision about my treatment." This unclear medical situation necessitates good communication between the patient and his significant other so that a good treatment decision can be arrived at.

When a family system is called upon to deal with a severely overwhelming situation such as a traumatic experience, coping skills are overloaded and the usual mechanisms break down, and the delicate balance—of the crucial ecology of relationships is threatened. Areas of communication that have been weak or faltering become magnified, just when their good functioning is most important.

We have discussed the importance of access to social support as a factor in the positive reemergence and healing of trauma. It has also been shown to be of value in both quality of life and life extension with breast cancer patient. We have no identical research with regard to prostate cancer patients, but both are hormone-driven cancers and both tend to respond to psychological interventions.

At a time of great difficulty like this, couples need each other's support. However, what we are confronting head on in this situation can be the worst aspect of dealing with the clash between male and female culture. As one professional whom we interviewed said, "Men share a dissociative relationship with their bodies, which is a disadvantage when they have a medical problem. The urogenital area is a particularly emotion-laden and taboo area, and they have much naïveté and ignorance about this area. They're not sure how their own bodies work, and when they are diagnosed and have surgery, they are frightened to find out where or what their urogenital area's purpose is. This is a culturally laden issue; the norm in our culture is for the women to know the subject of inner bodily workings and to assess it—but men don't" (Litwin, Personal communication, 1993). But men have difficulty in sharing this need with women. Traditional male development stresses the need to find solutions and to find them by themselves. Prostate cancer may make men feel as if they have no solutions, and they may often retreat into themselves. So, we have two people, possibly feeling the same thing, often unable to reach out and touch each other to help make themselves feel better.

What both members of the couple share is a wish that this thing had never happened, together with a terror of what its future may hold. Beyond that, they wish that they had some way of finding a road map through this mess. What they need, more than anything else, is support from each other. But because they are each in their own traumatic state, and because this particular state can create a terrible sense of inadequacy in men, they may find themselves each alone, like two terrified and frozen strangers.

What about the woman's needs? Jean Baker Miller, Carol Gilligan, and others have taught us that women's psychological development and well being are based on connectedness. Therefore, isolation makes them feel desolate. With prostate cancer, men feel desolate, too, because they feel cut off for their sense of their sexual selves and question whether they have any other means of connecting. One of the women we interviewed told us, "Before the diagnosis, we were both active, but different. I was more of a people person. He was more contemplative and less gregarious. Our relationship was not ideal because of our differences and troubles in communicating. Our best area of communication was sex." With sexuality questioned and frequently disturbed by this disease, how can men and women help each other?

Over and over again in our interviews, women described their partners' reaction to the diagnosis as shock and fear—but mostly, they withdrew. The women felt themselves left alone with their own fears, wishing to be able to do the traditional female job of comforting and nurturing and attempting to ameliorate the situation. Instead, they were alone. John Gray, in his book, *Men Are from Mars, Women Are From Venus* (1992), talks about how women need to talk things out to understand what they feel, but men need to retreat in silence—to go into their cave. For men, the only way to find solutions is to go to a place where no one else is permitted in and just mull it through until it's worked out. A "cave" can be a silent place in a room with his partner, in another room, or in a runaway place.

Knowing what we do about women and connectedness, we can understand that when a man is silent, he becomes a projection screen for everything the woman is feeling about herself—for example, "Why didn't I get him to the doctor earlier," or "I bet he blames me for his cancer," or "I should have let him come home from the hospital when he wanted to and not when I thought it would be best," or the ultimate fear, "He probably should have married Mary Jane, and then he'd never have gotten sick."

Another unique aspect of prostate cancer is the fallout of the response to the initial impact of diagnosis. Having lost the magical thinking that made them feel invincible and invulnerable, and accepted that they do have cancer, they now reconstruct that bubble and try to believe that, although they are warned about side effects of treatment, these happen to other men, but not to them. A large portion of the men whom we interviewed had an understandable initial reaction of "do whatever it takes to get the cancer out of me and make sure that it's all gone."

But studies of the quality of life of posttreatment prostate cancer patients done by Dr. Mark Litwin at UCLA (Personal communication, 1993) has shown that all choices yield important side effects that can range from being simply annoying to having a dreadful effect on the patient, as well as on his partner's quality of life.

Imagine the experience of a man in his 50s, 60s, or 70s who is suddenly infantilized by incontinence and forced to wear a diaper or a pad, or experiment with a number of contraptions and treatments for a function he thought he had conquered at the age of 2! Imagine, as well, the experience of a man who has been raised to define his masculinity by his sexual prowess, suddenly reduced to impotence! Their reactions are withdrawal, flight, anger, frustration, and others, but they are rarely shared in open discussion with their partners.

Should you think we are exaggerating, when we first discussed our project with Pat Turcillo, the nurse who coordinates the UCLA Prostate Program (Personal communication, 1993), she immediately gave us a long list of women who, she said, "Were dying to talk to someone about their experience. These women are so angry," she said, "because their men refused to talk about their distress, and because they were reluctant to experiment with other ways of expressing sexuality." Like the woman we quoted earlier, many men use sexuality as their major emotional expression. Without it, the women felt abandoned. When we interviewed these women, we needed about four times the usual interview time because, as one woman said, "Forgive me for blabbing so much, but there's no one else I can tell about this." Spouses attend the support group meetings with the patients, but as several told us, "We discuss the issues but not the feelings." Others told us that whatever was discussed at the meeting was simply left there and not carried home.

Besides the anger, frustration, fear, and terror, perhaps the most apparent issues for these couples are loneliness and isolation. Having inadequate support and difficulties in communication, this should not be surprising. One 65-year-old patient said, "I felt as if I'd somehow, accidentally, been transported to some other planet, and that no one around me could possibly understand, much less appreciate, what I was going through." And the 60-year-old wife of a patient said, "I went from being part of a couple to being less than a single person. It was like being a kid who's lost. I wanted to cry out for help, for attention, for someone to take care of me. But as an adult, and especially as an adult having to be strong in a terrifying situation like this one, I just couldn't let myself do that."

When a recurrence or metastasis occurs, it reawakens all of the old fears and psychological needs and is further aggravated by a sense of failure and loss of hope.

ENDING TREATMENT

The end of cancer treatment is an often overlooked but crucial point. The patient reemerges from an environment where he or she may have been surrounded by others who have shared a sense of having been understood. She is then suddenly catapulted in the real world, where people in her surroundings have not shared any of her experience, and she may feel a sense of alienation and loneliness that is aggravated by a lack of understanding. She may find that those who have not shared her experience are trying to deny their own fears and want her to forget about her illness and make it disappear. The role of the therapist is crucial here, as well.

Palliative Care and Facing Death

Palliative care may be an area rarely seen as a part of your work. People in this situation are aware that they have a life-threatening illness for which there is little more that can be done medically. It is a time to help patients review their life experience, deal with unfinished business, or talk about whatever pains or joys that come to their mind. It is a time to ease the fears of facing death and to help to complete a focus on the positive aspects of their lives.

All of this may feel frightening and overwhelming both to the practitioner who deals with it and to the patient. Arthur Kleinman says, "Nothing so concentrates experience and clarifies the central conditions of living as serious illness" (Personal communication, 1998).

Dr. Balfour Mount, one of the founders of the palliative care movement and creator of the Palliative Care Centre of McGill University's Royal Victoria Hospital, tells us that "I have come to view life as a search for meaning, purpose, and personal connection to something greater and more enduring than the self. . . . The quest is really about connectedness, whether to one's belief system, family, or to self. Our intactness as persons comes not from the intactness of body but from the wholeness in the web of relationships" (Personal communication, 2000).

Palliative care strives to provide an opportunity for the dying patient to complete and maintain that wholeness and provide a sense of peace as he or she faces death. It allows the patient to talk about dying and to create a sense of completion for himself. An opportunity for life review is central to the experience. A sign in the Palliative Care center of a Montreal hospital reads, "We are here. We will be with you in your living and your dying. We will free you from pain and give you the freedom to find your own meaning in your life, your way. We will comfort you and those you love, not always with words, often with a touch or a glance. We will bring you hope not for tomorrow but for this day. We will not leave you. We will watch with you. We will be there" (Quoted by D. Nebenzahl, the *Montreal Gazette,* April 20, 2004). Some of my students and colleagues have found that working or volunteering in palliative care settings is one of the most fulfilling professional experiences that they have had. It is an aspect of trauma that has often been overlooked in our work and one with which we should become more familiar.

This chapter has focused on traumas that many of us may overlook, simply because they attack us from within ourselves. Yet these are probably responsible for more deaths than we usually associate with trauma experiences.

It is extremely important for mental heath practitioners to be aware of all aspects of the cancer experience and its impact on patients and others, so that we can apply our skills in dealing with this prevalent and destructive trauma.

REFERENCES

Buber, M. (1958). *I and thou.* New York: Scribner.

Cunningham, A. J. (2000). *The healing journey.* Toronto: Key Porter Books.

Gilligan, C. (1982). *In a different voice.* Cambridge, MA: Harvard University Press.

Gray, J. (1992). *Men are from Mars, women are from Venus.* New York: Harper Collins Publishers.

Green, B. L., Rowland, J. H., Krupnick, J. L., Epstein, S. A., Stockton, P., Spertus, I., et al. (1998). Prevalence of posttraumatic stress disorder in women with breast cancer. *Psychosomatics, 35,* 102–111.

Haber, S., Wainrib, B., Acuff, C., Goodheart, C., Mikesell, S., Ayers, L., et al. (1993). *Breast cancer: A psychological treatment manual, Division 42.* Washington, DC: American Psychological Association.

Koopman, C., Butler, L. D., Classen, C. Giese-Davis, J., et al. (2002). Traumatic stress symptoms among women with recently diagnosed primary breast cancer. *Journal of Traumatic Stress, 15*(4), 277–287.

Lerner, M. (1994). *Choices in healing.* Cambridge, MA: The MIT Press.

Miller, J. B. (1972). *Towards a new psychology of women.* Boston: Beacon Press.

Nebenzahl, D. (2004, April 20). The *Montreal Gazette.*

Parad, H. J. (1965). *Crisis intervention: Selected readings.* Milwaukee, WI: Family Service Associate of America.

Parad, H. T., & Parad, L. G. (1990). *Crisis intervention, Book 2.* Milwaukee, WI: New York Family Service Association of America.

Puryear, D. A. (1979). *Helping people in crisis.* San Francisco: Jossy-Bass.

Rollin, B. (1976). *First you cry.* Baltimore, MD: Lippincott.

Shneidman, E. (1985). *Definition of suicide.* New York: Wiley.

Thomas, L. (1974). *Lives of a cell: Notes of a biology watcher.* New York: Viking.

Van Gennep, A. (1960). *Rites of passage.* Chicago: University of Chicago Press.

Wainrib, B. (1975). On oppression, support and the "Phoenix Phenomenon". Unpublished doctoral paper, University of Massachusetts, Amherst, MA.

Wainrib, B. (1998). In B. Wainrib & E. Bloch, *Crisis intervention and trauma response, theory and practice.* New York: Springer Publishing.

CHAPTER 6

Resilience and the Phoenix Phenomenon

The world breaks everyone, and afterward, some grow strong at the broken places.

—Ernest Hemingway (1929)

THE "PHOENIX PHENOMENON"

When we meet and work with people who have been through traumatic situations, we can not automatically assume that they have been irrevocably injured emotionally and psychologically. Trauma, like any other aspect of human existence, is not a "one size fits all" experience. Some will respond to traumatic situations with severe psychological damage, but others will manifest a sense of resilience or hardiness, and it is our job to watch for these strengths and to help the client to build upon them.

We need to understand, however, how these strengths develop and how they can be manifest. Anthony and Cohler (1987) remind us that "The emphasis on deficit and maldevelopment in psyche has largely remained, following the example of medicine's emphasis in disease. But recently, there has been a movement in psychology to conceptualize human nature in terms of strengths and abilities not as weaknesses and deficiencies" (Anthony & Cohler, 1987).

At the header of this chapter, I quoted from Ernest Hemingway's novel *A Farewell to Arms*. Growing "strong at the broken places" has been a fascination of mine for many years. Understanding what makes some people become "phoenixes"—that is, what makes them grow strong at the broken places, and what makes others "victims" as a result of trauma has been at the root of this interest. In my previous book, I wrote the following:

> Our own experiences with the lives of clients, as well as our own life, has led us to the concept of the Phoenix Phenomenon, which is the ultimate goal of empowerment. The phoenix, as you may recall, was a mythic bird that had the capacity to resurrect itself, to rise, at it were, from its own ashes. Our work has shown that the impact of life crisis or trauma can provoke either a positive or negative response which has the potential for change (Wainrib, in Wainrib & Bloch, 1998).

PHOENIXES AMONGST US

Senator Max Clelland's Story

We strongly recommend to all readers the viewing of a video called *Strong at the Broken Places* (Cambridge Documentary Films, Inc., 1998). The video presents biographical stories about four extremely traumatized people who have not only survived but who have used their experience to make important contributions to humanity.

In writing about the concept of resilience as shown by the four protagonists seen in the film, Dr. Susan Pauker (1998) of Harvard Medical School and the Harvard Pilgrim Health Care Foundation, reports the following:

> Most (North) Americans have not personally suffered through war. Yet all of us have endured some form of trauma to our souls. Our parents were human and, therefore, imperfect. Harsh words, a back hand to the rump, a cry of "stupid" or "lazy!" have crushed our spirits and limited our horizons. School bullies, test scores, temptations of drugs or sex, illness, poverty and man's inhumanity to man have all left us with broken spots. Like damaged DNA, these fractures get passed on to the next generation, aided by alcohol, addictions, negative societal and parental role models.

Pauker (1998) continues,

> The job for all of us is to crash through the cycle of violence, choose to heal ourselves from our vast or minor injuries, access love and support around us, arise, and correct for our children and others the very circumstances which tried our own spirits and from which we now can draw strength.

Describing the characters in this film, Dr. Pauker says,

> four humans, severely traumatized by life's circumstances, choose to turn away from grief and pain and head toward healing. They could not control the circumstances of their trauma, but they chose to control their responses. From the point, deeper in despair than most of us can imagine surviving, the featured speakers turned, arose, and chose a life of strength. Having accessed love, or laughter, or constant kindness, they chose to mend at their broken places. This healing took the form in each case of giving back, of helping to fix the societal ills from which they had almost died spiritually.

One of the most moving examples in this video is the experience of Max Clelland, who was left for dead in Vietnam, eventually rescued having lost three of his limbs.

Those of us who watched the Democratic National Committee presidential nominations saw and heard Clelland's moving presentation, and have seen or read about his remarkable accomplishments after his Vietnam experience.

Clelland has said, "The worst thing I could have done at the twenty six, missing an arm and two legs was to sit in a corner of my mother's living room and do nothing."

He is a gifted, outstanding example of one of the most resilient people amongst us, a true phoenix. But it does not require that unusual quality of pain to become a "phoenix," as we will see in the following sections.

John's Story

My student John waited to talk to me one evening after our graduate trauma class. He is a very bright man who was the principal of a school for students who, for a variety of reasons, had been expelled from other schools. He, however, saw these students not as failures but as young people who needed a different approach to their work and their life. He has been extremely successful with his graduates. In his class presentation, he described his work in this area as a "Bridge Over Troubled Waters" and described a host of creative, supportive techniques he had devised to encourage the healthy, positive aspects of his students. That evening, however, he wanted to tell me about the death of his brother.

John came from a large family, and each child was quite industrious at a young age. An older brother had a paper route. One morning, while delivering papers at the age of 12, his brother was murdered. Although this event occurred over 20 years previously, no one has been able to find the perpetrator. Understandably, the entire family was thrown into traumatic shock. And, one by one, the trauma turned into growth and change as each family member, from the father to the youngest child, recreated their lives by redirecting their goals to focus on professions that helped other people.

John's chosen profession was typical. Of the others, one became a nurse, one a social worker, one a psychologist, and others in helping professions, and so on. John would pick hurt and emotionally injured children and create an environment for them in which they could not only live but flourish.

Painful as this experience had been, John and his family redirected their anguish into a direction of both healing and growth; they are examples of the Phoenix Phenomenon. John is not only a phoenix himself, but, in a beautifully creative manner, he touches the lives of many, directing them toward strength and success.

Jeff's Story

I was standing on line at a supermarket one day when I glanced down at one of those tabloids that adorn the check-outs. This one, however caught my eye. The headline said "Unluckiest Man in America is the Happiest." I looked at the picture of this "unluckiest" man and saw that it was Jeff, a young man that I had known all of his life. There he was, walking along the beach in Malibu, California, with his three-legged dog. I knew that the dog had been rescued from the pound, subsequently rear-ended by a hit and run car, and saved by Jeff despite its loss of a leg and its consequent incontinence.

Jeff had been a delightful and somewhat difficult little boy. His parents report that he was that way even before birth and that he had tangled himself up so totally in his umbilical cord that it was a mere act of luck that he was delivered quickly by induction, with the umbilical cord wrapped around his neck several times. The effect of this defect was to facilitate his becoming a rather rambunctious but fearless child. When it was discovered that he could not walk because his heel cords were elongated, at the age of a year and a half, his legs were put into casts from the toes to the knees. His reaction to this was the first indication of what was to come throughout his life: He quickly learned that if he climbed up on a chair and then onto the table, he could jump off, break the casts, and be free for a few days before they were replaced.

The birth defect made traditional schooling difficult for him. His verbal acuity was extremely high, but he was somewhat hyperactive and had difficulty following through with written work. Nevertheless, he went into the world with a very bright mind and the ability to charm anyone. And he was constantly testing himself to the limits: becoming a black belt in Kung Fu, a long distance runner, a triathlete, and a charming raconteur.

Eventually he ended up living in California, and through a rather roundabout way, he found himself in the restaurant business, where his charm and sparkling verbal acuity made him a winner. However, the world was about to test him, landing him on that newspaper cover. The first thing that happened was that his restaurant was destroyed during the Los Angeles riots. Somehow he recovered from this and was busy building an equally interesting new restaurant on the beach. In his glory days, he bought a house on top of the mountains in Malibu, overlooking the ocean. Shortly after he moved into it, wild fires struck that area and destroyed his house. In his true fashion, he stayed with the house trying to protect it to the end. He slid down the mountainside, picking up an elderly woman as he came down, and finally got to a safe place. He was subsequently to learn that in the course of this disaster, his insurance company went into bankruptcy. His parents reported that his reaction to that was simply to focus on the fact that he still had his new restaurant and a place to live—a little hut on the beach. But not long after that experience, the earthquake hit and destroyed his precious new restaurant. And not much later, a major storm hit and washed away his safe place on the beach. If I did not know this young man personally, I would have suspected that some of this was fiction, but unfortunately, it was real.

One of Jeff's great strengths was his ability to create significant support systems around him. Articulate and fun to be with, he attracted people easily. He was also considerate, and when he heard about the earthquake, his first reaction was to make sure that his entire community had adequate drinking water before he took care of his own needs. He was interviewed for television's *Inside Edition* program, where he told the interviewer, "I had the misfortune of being in the wrong place at the wrong time, three times. . . . I'm the luckiest guy you're ever going to meet. We are standing here and we are talking about it. We regroup and take on the world" (*Inside Edition,* 1993).

CREATING RESILIENCE

There is considerable research about what contributes to creating resilience, a capacity held by some individuals to respond positively to life's difficulties, crises, and traumas. "For some people, trauma and loss actually facilitate a move toward health" (Card 1983, Sledge et al., 1980, p. 83). A traumatic incident can become the center around which a victim reorganizes a previously disorganized life, reorienting values and goals (Ursano, 1981).

John and Jeff and Senator Clelland are examples of people who have been able to create and access support mechanisms in time of trauma and use them for both their and others' needs. These mechanisms may be internal, external, or both.

Increasing information that points to the physiological components of resilience has been developed in the recent past. In an article by Southwick, Morgan, Vythilingam, Krystal, and Charney (2003), the authors find that "neurobiological factors that potentially convey protection and/or promote resilience in the face of stress and trauma" are currently receiving more and more attention.

> By studying animals and humans who have adapted well to highly adverse conditions researchers have recently begun to identify a neurochemical profile that characterizes resilient individuals and that may, in the future help to predict who will develop psychiatric symptoms in response to traumatic stress and who will rebound rapidly or even benefit from their challenging experiences." The factors that seem to be most helpful in these various approaches to research all center around the "emerging neurobiology of resilience" (Charney, in Vythilingam, Krystal, and Charney, 2003, p. 37).
>
> Southwick, and colleagues report that during situations of danger, the sympathetic nervous system (SNS) releases epinephrine and norepinephrines in order to protect the organism. The magnitude of sympathetic nervous system responses to stress and danger varies from one person to the next. Some people have an unusually robust SNS response to stress and in essence "over-react."
>
> Unchecked persistent SNS hyper-responsiveness may contribute to chronic anxiety, hypervigilance, fear, intrusive memories, and increased risk for hypertension and cardiovascular disease. Such responses have been found in individuals with PTSD (Southwick et al., 2003).

In contrast, it is likely that psychologically resilient individuals maintain SNS activation within a window of adaptive elevation, high enough to respond to danger but not so high as to produce incapacity, anxiety and fear (Charney, 2003).

The authors have positive expectations of greater understanding of the neurobiological aspect of resilience and expect it will lead to prevention and/or improved treatment of stress related disorders such as PTSD. A particularly interesting aspect of their research suggests that "antidepressants have shown to protect against effects of stress in animals and to stimulate the re-growth of hippocampal neurons (critical for learning and memory) that have been damaged by stress." Their findings also reinforce our original concepts in this area, that "some forms of psychotherapy and social support may serve to bolster extinction of the fear-conditioned memories and cortical inhibition of limbic hyper-responsivity so commonly seen in individuals with anxiety disorder" (Charney, 2003). As we will see in the next section, this information has now come full circle from my own thinking which originated in the 1970s.

We have gone from the initial concept of the importance of support to the more recent neurological information and back again to human support.

What Creates a Phoenix?

My initial description and writing about the Phoenix Phenomenon was in a paper I wrote in my doctoral program in 1975. The paper was called "On Oppression, Support and the 'Phoenix Phenomenon.'" Unfortunately, I did not attempt to have it published, and I have recently seen a book that uses the term that I thought I had created! My hypothesis at that time was the concept of the oppression/support ratio. This ratio relates to the degree to which an individual has a balance of social support appropriate to his or her needs at a time of crisis. In theory, this balance will help that person have sufficient emotional strength to overcome oppression, pain, trauma, and other aspects of life's difficulties. Beyond that work, my experience had been that not only would these people survive the experience but that often, very difficult experiences would become springboards to enhance psychological growth, hence the image of the phoenix rising.

"Support" was defined as "access to and experience of the quality of relationship appropriate to the specific need at the time." In order to further define and expand this concept in my 1975 doctoral thesis, "A Tri-Level Model of Human Support and Its Applications," I defined three levels of support. They are the following:

Level I. Contact

Defined as "that minimal face to face relationship between individuals as they move within each other's orbit during the course of their waking hours: the elementary social behavior which occurs when two or more people recognize the existence of each other and confirm the focal person's place in the system or situation."

Level 2. Social/Functional Relationships

These relationships assume a history or the creation of one and are often found and legitimized by work or play situations which have a circumscribed parameter. They create an experience of complementary and mutual respect with the goal of companionship/friendship in sharing external experiences.

Level 3. Validation Relationships

These are defined as "a relationship which recognizes the core of one's existence as a unique individual," such as those defined by Buber: "that when he met me he really met me . . . that he opened his eyes and saw who I was. That he did not confuse me with anyone else" (Buber, 1958).

This is of course a simplification of the elements involved in what could provide an individual with the possibility of sufficient resilience to snap back from some of life's horrors. Research also indicates that adequate social support may function to protect victims of crisis from both physical and mental disorder (Gavayla, 1987). Coates in *Trauma and Human Bonds* (2003) tells us that

> the greater the strength of the human bonds that connect an individual to others and the more those bonds are accessible in times of danger, the less likely it is that an individual will be severely traumatized and the more likely it is that he or she may recover afterward. There is a limit, to be sure, that even the most securely related individual will be overwhelmed by a threat that is massive to be borne whether it occurs in war or on the 96th floor of a burning building. But one must also remember that the basic human instinct, even on the 96th floor, is to make contact with someone else, even if it has to be by cell phone and even when it is clear that it will be futile in terms of rescue (p. 4).

For people with limited support systems, disaster support groups can be helpful. Groups help to counter isolation, challenge erroneous beliefs about uniqueness and pathology, provide emotional support, and allow survivors to share concrete information and recovery tips (Grossman, 1973). Mental health staff may be involved in setting up self-help support groups for survivors or may facilitate support groups.

In dealing with trauma, crisis, or other major difficulties, we often ask ourselves how some people can experience horrible, traumatic life experiences and emerge from them able to grow and change and have a positive impact on others. Part of the process is that the crisis makes one reassess one's life. Some people may find at this junction, that they are really content with their life as it was before the crisis and that they cherish that. These people will do their best to reconstruct their life in the same format after the trauma. This may, however, not always be possible. The circumstances of the crisis or trauma, whether it be loss of a loved one, a life-threatening illness, or the destruction of one's home, may make the "make it the way it used to be" wish just that. These people may need support and direction in reconstructing their lives, even if they would like them to proceed as they had been before the event. For others, however, the crisis will magnify those elements in their life which have been causing them subliminal distress, which may have previously been unacknowledged. For those people, given the right combination of resources, the crisis can become a medium to new growth.

A recent article by Bonanno (2004) informs us that "Resilience reflects the ability to maintain a stable equilibrium of . . . protective factors that foster the development of positive outcomes and healthy personality characteristics among children exposed to unfavorable or aversive life circumstances" (p. 20). "Resilient individuals . . . generally exhibit a stable trajectory of healthy functioning across time as well as the capacity for generative experiences and positive emotions"(Bonanno, Papa, & O'Neil, 2001).

Other research on resilience is being done by Dr. Mark Chesler at the University of Michigan, with his colleagues Dr. Bradley Zebrack of the University of Southern California and D. Carla Parry of the University of Colorado Health Sciences Center. This group uses the term "posttraumatic growth," which they feel is somewhat different from "resilience." They define Posttraumatic Growth as "The experience of expression of positive life change as an outcome of a trauma or life crisis, . . . of having 'something good' come out of difficult situations."

Frankly, I see little difference between this, my concept of the Phoenix Phenomenon, and other colleagues' identifications, and I respect their position. They tell us that they can identify this change when informants attribute growth or change in their lives as a result of the trauma, which I fully support. Working with survivors of childhood cancer, Chesler has identified growth in the following areas:

- New and greater strength (psychological toughness/ resilience).
- Greater compassion and empathy for others who have illness/ disabilities.
- Greater psychological/emotional maturity.

- A recognition of the vulnerability and struggle and a deeper appreciation for life.
- New values in life priorities (often not materialistic heightened intimacy in relationships)
- Greater existential and spiritual clarity (who am I, what is my purpose in life, etc.)

He adds "It make sense to theorize posttraumatic growth." One of the aspects he has identified is "the support from significant others who can provide love, a hopeful message, and a supportive story of their illness experience." This reflects our model of the original Phoenix Phenomenon (Chesler, 2003).

An organization that may be of more help to clients than practitioners is ResilienceNet. They define resilience as the "human capacity and ability to face, overcome, be strengthened by, and even be transformed by experiences of adversity."

They describe themselves:

> ResilienceNet brings together information available through the Internet and conventional published sources about the development and expression of human resilience. Although we endeavor to cover all aspects of resilience, ResilienceNet focuses on resilience in children, youth, and families. Additional topics, especially as they impact on children, youth, and families, are included as well, such as
>
> - resilience of communities resilience and life-long physical and mental health
> - resilience related to culture, ethnicity, and gender
> - children and adults at risk

ResilienceNet provides information about resilience in the following forms: Comprehensive bibliographies of the resilience literature, drawn from psychology, education, medicine, and relevant articles and descriptions of programs found in the popular literature; and descriptions of and links to Web sites containing information about resilience.

There is a far greater interest in this aspect of trauma than there has been in the past, and the reader is encouraged to keep up with the current work through the use of the internet as well as professional journals. What was once mere speculation has now become a major interest. While we may never find a single theory that can account for the diversity of experiences and life background that certainly must feed into adult resilience, we can search for answers. Some of these include the work of Anthony and Cohler

(1987), who have studied invulnerable children. They found that these invulnerable children seem somehow to rise to and often perform better than ever in the face of adversity. Their developmental histories are characterized by a certain temperamental robustness that is apparent even in infancy, coupled with strong "in-the-world" feelings and attitudes. They seem inherently endowed with a wide range of competencies, and their normal defenses, coping skills, and creativity grow with age. Their relationships are soundly based and enduring. They are interpersonally skillful, popular with other children and adults, well regarded by themselves and others, assertive on their own behalf, have a strong sense of personal control, and take responsibility for their own actions. They are reflective, rather than impulsive, show a healthy creativity, and keep a good hold on their emotions, although they are capable of experiencing and expressing a full range of normal feelings. Their eagerness to learn, their curiosity, and their absorption with scholastic subjects endear them to teachers, so that school is often a place of refuge, support, and encouragement. In dealing with stresses or potentially traumatic experiences, these resilient children demonstrate higher and better focused intelligence, use more divergent or creative thinking in approaching problems, show an increased capacity to select out the particular aspects of adversity required to overcome, and make greater use of goal-oriented strategies to plan the necessary steps to solve the problem without becoming overwhelmed by the complexity or hopelessness of the situation (Anthony & Cohler, in Miller, 1998).

What do we know about children who grow up with less stable families? Miller (1998) further reports on Cohler's work, saying that

> according to Cohler (1987), a fortunate minority of the children of psychiatrically ill parents are better able to cope with the adversity of unreliable and often emotionally inaccessible caretakers because they have greater innate ego strength, creative abilities, and increased personal and physical attractiveness. Such traits enable these children to continue to reach out successfully to others inside and outside the family for support.

Miller goes on to say that "to the extent that their parents are able to provide basic care and assistance, these resilient children appear to be successful in engaging the parents. When a disturbed parent is not accessible, these children are able to seek out alternative providers of adult care, turning to such available adults as relatives, teachers, and family friends." Rutter (1985), however, may be on to a larger part of the question; he has observed that children reared by seriously mentally ill parents may cope by separating themselves emotionally from their homes and developing their ties elsewhere. Others become resilient by taking on responsibilities for coping with stress in the family situation and doing so successfully.

Anthony also suggested that "Developing a philosophy of life or a religious outlook may also be highly effective in fostering and supporting resilience" (1974). We will reconsider this issue in a later chapter.

Many researchers have tried to isolate resilient people directly after a traumatic experience. For example, Macmillan, Smith, and Fisher (1997) (in Miller [1998]) studied people at the end of three major traumas: a tornado, a plane crash, and a mass shooting. They interviewed survivors 4 to 6 weeks after each incident and then again 3 years later. They found those survivors "who perceived a benefit from the disaster at the initial interview were found to have better post traumatic adjustment 3 years later." What kinds of things could constitute "benefits" from such disaster? They reported increased personal closeness with others, increased cohesion of the overall community, a greater sense of personal growth, and material gain.

Murphy and Moriarty (1976) tell us that "Most adaptive, resilient children don't have to go it alone. Many are lucky enough to have a nurturing home environment that reinforces their own strong character traits. They also noted that many of the parents of children who cope well are good copers themselves and provide models of resilience to their children. Parents who cope well have a distinctive profile: they enjoy their children, provide them with a facilitating environment without stepping on their autonomy, support their efforts to care for themselves, furnish a reassuring background, and are highly receptive to their ideas and creative expressions" (Miller 1998, p. 278). True coping, in this view, employs many more ego skills than are required for purely defensive purposes.

Coping mechanisms differ from defense mechanisms in being more flexible, purposive, selective, oriented toward present relative and future planning, involving largely conscious, reality-based thinking, and coordinating individual needs with external reality. While defense usually needs to be worked through in formal therapy, Anthony (in Anthony & Cohler, 1987) notes, coping is a learnable skill, which also means that parents and teachers, as well as therapists, can serve as appropriate models.

TOUGHNESS AND HARDINESS

As we have seen, the gamut of concepts of understanding and attempting to create resilience runs from psychobiological theory to behavioral learnings.

Miller (1998) quotes Dienstbier's model which is based upon cortex responses to stressful challenges. He defines the nature of the toughness trait:
"The trait variable of toughness is seen as a buffer against the health-debilitating effects of stressful life events. Toughness is defined as a distinct reaction pattern to stress, mental or physical, that characterizes animals and humans who cope effectively. . . ." Apparently humans are not distinct in the ownership of this trait. Animal, as well as human research, has shown that: "Bodily response of individuals high in the toughness trait differs dramatically from that of individuals low in toughness. In tough subjects, the normal, baseline activity in the two systems is relatively low, indicating that tough organisms are at relative ease under ordinary circumstances." These characteristics appear to manifest themselves primarily in situations of stress. Apparently the process, at this time according to Diestenbier, is that

> the sympathetic nervous system-adrenal medulla system springs into action quickly and efficiently, while the pituitary-adrenal cortex system remains relatively stable. As soon as the emergency is over, the adrenaline response abates quickly to baseline, while the cortisol response remains low. It is thus the smoothness and efficiency of the physiological arousal pattern that characterizes the toughness response (Dienstbier, 1989).

So-called "non-tough" reactors show a different pattern. "By contrast," Dienstbier has found, "the physiological reaction of 'non-toughs' tends to be more exaggerated and long-lasting; further, this reaction occurs not just to dire emergencies but to everyday hassles. The adrenaline rush is greater and stays higher longer, while cortisol levels are also elevated." Apparently, the effect of this function is that "The result is greater, more disorganizing arousal, less effective coping, and faster."

Thus, Dienstbier's (1989) conceptualization leaves room for therapeutic intervention. "According to the model, the physiological toughness response, or its absence interacts with a person's psychological appraisal of his own ability to cope with challenge. This, in turn, contributes to the person's self-image as an effective master of adversity or, alternatively, as a helpless reactor." It is not surprising then, that having experienced this successful response to stress, future experiences will be more easily dealt with.

Dienstbier concludes,

> In this conceptualization, the most effective place to intervene would be at the psychological level. Learning effective coping skills can render the physiological reaction of the two systems to threat or challenge less intense and more automatic. Instead of being immobilized by uncertainty

or panic, for example, the person can be stimulated by the nervous system's appraisal of threat to seek out adaptive solutions" (Dienstbier, 1989, quoted in Miller, 1998).

In the January 2004 edition of the *American Psychologist*, Bonanno gives us an interesting article titled "Loss, Trauma and Resilience." In reviewing concepts that have been developed in this area, he describes the concept of "hardiness." Developed by Kobassa, Maddi, and Kahn in 1982, "Hardiness" is described as

consisting of three dimensions: being committed to finding meaningful purpose in life, the belief that one can influence one's surroundings and the outcome of events, and the belief that one can learn and grow from both positive and negative life experiences. Armed with this set of beliefs, hardy individuals have been found to appraise potentially stressful situations as less threatening, thus minimizing the experience of distress. Hardy individuals are also more confident and better able to use active coping and social support, thus helping them deal with the distress they do experience.

This concept can easily be applied to the experiences of John and Jeff that I described previously.

POSITIVE CHANGE FOLLOWING TRAUMA

Linley and Joseph, in an article titled "Positive Change Following Trauma and Adversity" (2004) report on

positive changes, following chronic illness, heart attacks, breast cancer, bone marrow transplants, HIV and AIDs, rape and sexual assault, military combat, maritime disasters, plane crashes tornadoes, shootings, bereavement, injury recovery from substance addiction and in the parents of children with disabilities. . . . These positive changes share the common factor of struggling with adversity (referred to) collectively as "adversarial growth" (pp. 11–21).

They also tell us that

from an applied perspective clinicians should be aware of the potential for positive change in their clients following trauma and adversity. Positive changes may be used as foundations for further therapeutic work providing hope that the trauma can be overcome (Calhoun & Tedeschi, 1999; Linley & Joseph, 2004) Interventions for post-traumatic stress disorder typically do not take account of the potential for adversarial growth (p. 12).

Greater levels of perceived threat and harm are associated with higher levels of adversarial growth. An interesting finding that reflects and validates our previously discussed section on the Phoenix Phenomenon is one that tells us that "social support satisfaction [is] positively associated with growth" (Linley & Joseph, 2004).

THE "SECOND DISASTER"

Although it would be ideal if any kind of trauma could be responded to in a manner that encouraged growth and development, some disasters perpetuate the opposite. Myers (1999) tells us about "the second disaster." She says contrary to creating positive experiences for survivors,

> the process of seeking help from government, voluntary agencies, and insurance companies is fraught with rules, red tape, hassles, delays, and disappointment for survivors of disaster. Feelings of helplessness and anger are common. Mental health staff may assist individuals by reassuring them that this "second disaster" "is a common phenomenon and that they are not alone in their frustration. Staff may need to help survivors find constructive channels for their anger that do not sabotage their efforts by alienating those trying to help them. (Myers, 1994)

There are also other types of "second disasters." For example, Antonucci (1985) indicated that "the presence of family support does not necessarily have a substantially positive impact, but its absence may be detrimental." A good example of this is the experience of a former student of mine. After she had been raped, rather than being given an appropriate caring response from her family she was, instead, shunned by them.

As we can expect, not every trauma ends up in a severe disaster. In some communities, mental health workers have participated in community organization activities, bringing individuals together at the neighborhood or community level to address concrete issues of concern. This process of community connection has assisted survivors with disaster recovery not only by helping with concrete problems, but by reestablishing feelings of control, competence, self-confidence, and effectiveness. Perhaps most important, the process helps to reestablish social bonds.

In fact, the idea that certain people naturally cope better with adversity than others, and thereby, suffer fewer ill-health effects has been articulated in a number of ways and supported by several lines of research. Kobasa (1979), Kobasa et al. (1982), Maddi (1990), and Maddi and Kobasa (1984) have proposed that the personality construct is a moderator in the stress-illness relationship. Hardiness is comprised of three main beliefs about the self and the world:

1. commitment: thinking of yourself and your environment as interesting and worthwhile and being able to find something constructive and meaningful in whatever you're doing.
2. control: believing that your own efforts can have an effect on what goes on around you.
3. challenge: believing that what improves your life is growth and learning rather than easy comfort and security. (Miller, 1998)

Benezra also studied survivors of Nazi persecution—people who coped well without professional intervention. But he too found that these people described a healthy secure upbringing characterized by a supportive relationship with their families, friends and others. After their traumatic incident, they were able to freely express feelings and talk about their trauma or to simply put it out of their minds and move on.

True coping, in this view, employs many more ego skills than are required for purely defensive purposes. Coping mechanisms differ from defense mechanisms in being more flexible, purposive, selective, oriented toward present reality and future planning, involving largely conscious, reality-based thinking, and coordinating individual needs with external reality. While defense usually needs to be worked through in formal therapy, Anthony (1987), quoted in Calhoun and Tedeschi (1999) notes, coping is a learnable skill, which also means that parents and teachers, as well as therapists, can serve as appropriate models.

PHOENIXES RISING FROM 9-11

As we have seen in so many traumatic situations, the September 11, 2001 (9-11) experience, horrible as it was, created its own set of "Phoenix" situations. My colleague, Dr. Pat Pitta, found that the impact of the 9-11 experience propelled her toward a reassessment of her own personal life. On September 12, she wrote the following:

> I have been doing a great deal of intervention and debriefing for my fellow neighbors. In Manhasset, where I live, there are many people who work in the financial district. We lost 33 lives in our town. In a neighboring town of Garden City, they lost 100 people and in Rockville Centre,

which is next to Garden City, another 50 people are dead. The loss here is overwhelming. People walk around in a daze. People seem gentler at the moment. I spoke to a congregation of 400 people in church on Wednesday evening, and it was the first time that a psychologist was invited to the altar to address the congregation. It was a moving experience (Personal communication, 2001).

Now, in addition to her busy psychotherapy practice, she is also a student in the ministry.

Each of us will respond in his or her own unique manner to traumatic situations. If we learn—and then are able to teach others—to recognize the "opportunity" as well as the "difficulty" in dealing with trauma, we help to facilitate more and more people to redirect their trauma experiences to new growth.

REFERENCES

Anthony, E. J. (1987). Risk, vulnerability and resilience: An overview. In E. J. Anthony & B. J. Cohler (Eds.), *The invulnerable child*. New York: Guilford Press.

Anthony, E. J.(1974). *The syndrome of the psychologically invulnerable child*. Quoted in E. J. Anthony & B. J. Cohler, (1987), *The invulnerable child*. New York: Guilford.

Anthony, E. J., & Cohler, B. J. (1987) *The invulnerable child*. New York: Guilford.

Anthony, E. J., & Cohler, B. J. (1998). In L. Miller (1998), *Shocks to the system: Psychotherapy of traumatic disability syndromes*. New York: W.W. Norton.

Antonucci, T. C. (1985). Personal characteristics, social support, and social behavior. In R. H. Binstock & E. Shanas (Eds.), *Handbook of aging and the social sciences* (pp. 94–128). New York: Van Nostrand Reinhold.

Benezra, E. E. (1996). Personality factors of individuals who survive traumatic experiences without professional help. *International Journal of Stress Management* 3, 147–153, quoted in Miller, (1998). *Shocks to the system* (p. 282). New York: Norton.

Bonanno, G. A. (2004). Loss, trauma, and human resilience. *American Psychologist, 59*(1), 20–28.

Bonanno, G. A., Papa, A., & O'Neil, K. (2001). Loss and human resilience. *Applied and Preventive Psychology, 10*, 193–206.

Buber, M. (1958). *I and thou*. New York: Scribner.

Calhoun, L. G., & Tedeschi, R. G. (1999). *Facilitating posttraumatic growth: A clinician's guide*. Mahwah, NJ: Lawrence Erlbaum Associates.

Card, J. J. (1983). *Lives after Viet Nam*. Lexington, MA: Lexington Books.

Chesler, M., Zebrack, B., & Parry, C. (2003[AU22]). *The Prevention Researcher, 10*(Suppl., December).

Coates, S. (2003). *Trauma and human bonds*. Hillsdale, New Jersey: The Analytic Press.

Dienstbier, R. A. (1989). Arousal and physiological toughness: Implications for mental and physical health. *Psychological Review, 96,* 84–100, quoted in L. Miller (1998), *Shocks to the system*. New York: Norton.

Gavayla, A. S. (1987). Reactions to the 1985 Mexican Earthquake: Case vignettes. *Hospital and Community Psychiatry, 38*(12), 1327–1330.

Grossman, L. (1973). Train crash: Social work and disaster services. *Social Work, 18*(5), 38–44.

Hemingway, E. (1929). *A farewell to arms*. New York: Charles Scribner's Sons.

Kobasa, S. C. (1979). Stressful life events, personality and health: An inquiry into hardiness. *Journal of Personality and Social Psychology, 37,* 1–11, quoted in Miller, (1998), *Shocks to the system*, 1–11. New York: Norton.

Kobasa, S. C., et al. (1982). The concept of hardiness: A brief but critical commentary. *Psychology, 37*(1), 1–11.

Kobasa, S. C., Maddi, S. R., & Kahn, S. (1982). Hardiness and health: A prospective study. *Journal of Personality and Social Pyschology, 42,* 168–177.

Lachman, C., & Young, B. (1993). Executive Producers, *Inside Edition*, "Earthquake Aftermath."

Linley, P. A., & Joseph, S. (2004). Positive change following trauma and adversity: An empirical review. *Journal of Traumatic Stress, 17*(1), 11–21.

MacMillan, Smith, & Fisher (1997), quoted in Miller, (1998), *Shocks to the system: Psychotherapy of traumatic disability syndromes* (p. 5). New York: W.W. Norton.

Maddi, S. R. (1990). Issues and interventions in stress mastery. In H. S. Friedman (Ed.), *Personality and disease*. New York: Wiley.

Maddi, S. R., & Kobasa, S. C. (1984). *The hardy executive: Health under stress*. Homewood, IL: Dow Jones-Irwin.

Miller, L. (1998). *Shocks to the system: Psychotherapy of traumatic disability syndromes,* (p. 281). New York: W.W. Norton.

Murphy, L., & Moriarty, A. (1976). *Perspectives on disaster recovery*. Norwalk, CT: Appleton-Century-Crofts.

Myers, D. (1999). In B. Hiley-Young (Ed.), *Disaster response and recovery: A handbook for mental health professionals*. National Center for Post-Traumatic Stress Disorder, Menlo Park, California.

Myers, D. (1994). Psychological recovery from disaster: Key concepts for delivery of mental health services. *NCP Clinical Quarterly, 4*(2).

Pauker, S. (1998). *September 11: Trauma and human bonds*. Hillsdale, New Jersey: The Analytic Press.

ResilienceNet. Retrieved from http://www.resiliencenet.com/

Rutter, M. (1985). Resilience in the face of adversity: Protective factors and resistance to psychiatric disorder. *British Journal of Psychiatry, 147,* 598–611.

Sledge, W. H., Boydston, J. A., & Rahe, A. J. (1980). Self-concept changes. *Archives of General Psychiatry, 37,* 43–44.

Southwick, S. M., Morgan, C. A.,Vythilingam, M., Krystal, J. H., & Charney, D. S. (2003). Emerging neurobiological factors in stress resilience. *PTSD Quarterly, 14*(4).

Strong at the Broken Places. (1998). Cambridge, MA: Documentary Films Inc.

Ursano, R. J. (1981). The Viet Nam era prisoner of war: Perceptivity, personality and development of psychiatric illness. *American Journal of Psychiatry, 138,* 315–318.

Wainrib, B. (1975). "On oppression, support and the 'Phoenix Phenomenon.'" Paper in partial fulfillment of doctoral requirements, University of Massachusetts, Amherst, MA.

Wainrib, B. (1998). In B. Wainrib & E. Bloch, *Crisis intervention and trauma response: Theory and practice.* New York: Springer Publishing.

CHAPTER 7

Trauma and the Mind

Traumatic events call into question basic human relationships. They breach the attachments of family, friendship, love and community. They shatter the construction of the self that is formed and sustained in relation to others.

—Judith Lewis Herman (1992)

EXPERIENCING TRAUMA: NEW ROOTS, OLD ROOTS

In the fall 2002 edition of *Spirituality and Health,* editor-in-chief Robert Scott relates a conversation he had with Archbishop Desmond Tutu of South Africa about the Archbishop's reactions to the September 11, 2001 (9-11) incident in America. Desmond Tutu is quoted as saying,

> I believe that one of the things that came out of 9-11 was realizing that you are vulnerable. . . . At the moment you don't know how to handle that because you are living with the illusion of being invincible. . . . Maybe just maybe Americans will realize that sense of insecurity as a daily fear of your sisters and brothers in other parts of the world . . . where (people) don't know from one moment to the next whether they're going to survive. . . . [In South Africa] that was a daily experience, this sense of insecurity, this sense of being fragile, that you are here today and gone tomorrow (Tutu, 2001).

As described previously, those of us who live in North America have certainly been fortunate in the limited number of mass traumas which we have experienced. Nevertheless, research findings from a nationally representative study indicated that over the life course, 10% of women and 5% of men in the United States experience PTSD (Kessler, Sonnega, Bromet, Hughes, & Nelson [1995], reported in Ozer and Weiss [2004]).

In chapter 4, I discussed issues of women and trauma. It is not surprising, then, to see that sexual assault is one of the most frequent types of traumas associated with PTSD in women. One out of every eight women experiences sexual assault during her lifetime.

Trauma evokes the preverbal experience of helplessness, the memory of which is stored in our spirits and our minds. It also has been shown to have an impact on our bodies. The experience of trauma changes an individual's sense of the world as well as his or her personal identity.

Before you read any further, take another moment or two to review your experiences during and after 9-11 and see how they may have changed your perception of security within your own life and your world. As well, think about any incidents in your life that may have felt like, or been diagnosed as "trauma." Think of your feelings in both mind and body at that time, and think of any similar feelings that you experienced after the trauma-stimulating situation. Reflect back for a few minutes on your 9-11 feelings and see if these were similar to those other feelings that you experienced. If you continue to have "flashbacks" or dreams or memories of the experience, note these as well. If you have had treatment for this condition, think back to what you felt was effective and what was not. As well, think back to your childhood and see if you can identify any traumatic memories that may have been related to your 9-11 experience.

For those of us who may experience difficulty in uncovering the source of a trauma in one of our patients, it may be of value to explore the patient's childhood. A study by Martin Teicher published in *Cerebrum* in 2000 demonstrated that "childhood abuse and neglect results in permanent physical changes to the developing human brain. These changes in brain structure appear to be significant enough to cause psychological and emotional problems in adulthood." Gaensbauer and Siegel (1995) has found that "Even prior to the onset of language fluency, symptomatology consistent with traditional posttraumatic diagnostic criteria can be observed. The developmental implications of early trauma, particularly if it is severe, appear to be significant." Indeed, childhood abuse is one of the most significant risk factors for traumatic reactions in adult women: Women who have experienced sexual assault in childhood are 2.5 to 3.1 times more likely to experience sexual assault in adulthood (Cloitrer, in Folette, [1998], p. 278). Gurvits et al. (1996) found that both women and men with chronic PTSD who had different kinds of traumatic events in their childhood demonstrated "neurological compromise," both in their history as well as in their physical examinations. Although an enormous amount of research on PTSD has been developed in the last decade or more, each piece of research makes us think that we have only scratched the surface of the impact of this extremely destructive experience.

Despite the relative peace of North America, we have found that: "In the U.S., 50% of women and 60% of men are exposed to at least one serious trauma during their lives. Individuals in developing nations are especially likely to be exposed to trauma and to multigenerational trauma: the repetitive exposure to individual, family, community and systemic violence and disaster" (ISTSS abstract, 2004).

In addition, individuals who have been exposed to trauma have been found to "have elevated rates of psychiatric disorders, including major depression, alcohol and drug dependence and PTSD. The negative impact of trauma extends beyond psychiatric morbidity and encompasses multiple realms, including functioning, quality of life and physical health" (ISTSS abstract, 2004).

Moreover, approximately half of adults have experienced a traumatic event. In a national survey of Vietnam veterans conducted in the late 1980s, Kulka et al. (1990) quoted in Weiss et al. (1992), estimated that "31% of males and 26% of females in this population had PTSD from their military service." Consider, then, what the overall numbers can be if we look at the global situation.

Some people demonstrate a somewhat unusual PTSD response. It is considered "partial PTSD" and appears to wax and wane. Life events after the PTSD experience may have little to do with it but can still set off the PTSD response. Weiss reports that these reactions are sometimes seen as "clinically significant symptoms of PTSD that do not meet the diagnostic criteria for the disorder." More than 830,000 Vietnam veterans who have manifested either "traditional PTSD" or "partial PTSD" have been found by Weiss et al. (1992) to demonstrate distress or impairment approximately 20 years after service.

Some research has identified a disparity between the 50% prevalence of exposure to trauma and the 7% lifetime prevalence of PTSD. This kind of data suggests, once again, that individual responses to trauma vary dramatically. This variability sparks what appears to be the key question in the field: Why do some people, and not others, develop PTSD? This issue has been of particular interest in recent years, leading to a search for systematic risk factors. Central questions have focused on the correlates or predictors that develop the disorder and the strength of these effects. Current conceptualizations of PTSD symptoms provide potential explanatory frameworks for appreciating how predictors may influence the stress response and lead to differential rates for PTSD. In a previous chapter, I identified an integration of newer concepts of resiliency that help us to understand its function.

Perhaps understanding why some people do and others do not respond positively to potentially traumatic situations is merely an extension of that work. Traumatic experiences can often be overlooked, particularly in populations that have been labeled with other diagnoses. Therefore, it is not surprising to find an article that reported that "43% of patients with severe mental illness fulfilled the criteria for PTSD but only 2% had this diagnosis in their charts." What seem to have emerged since the inclusion of trauma in the DSM (Diagnostic Statistical Manual—published annually by the American Psychiatric Association, "providing diagnostic criteria to improve the reliability of diagnostic judgment") are two schools of thought: those who rush to diagnose trauma and those who try to overlook it.

Others report that, regardless of the source of the trauma, depression and PTSD are interwoven disorders. Deering and colleagues (2002) conclude that "PTSD rarely appears as a singular disorder at any point in its course but is frequently accompanied by other manifestations of psychopathology" (pp. 219–232).

Importance of Early Assessment for PTSD

The International Society for Traumatic Stress Studies (ISTSS) has published a volume on Effective Treatments for PTSD that provides us with a rich overview of assessment tools for trauma. These include

- Structured Clinical Interview for DSM
- Revised Anxiety Disorders Scale
- PTSD Interview
- Clinician Administered PTSD Scales
- PTSD Symptom Scale Interview

In an addition to these, they include the Recommendations from the NIMH National Center for PTSD Conference on Assessment Standardization. These findings include the following:

- Clinical Interview: Structured diagnostic interviews provide valuable clinical information. Clinicians should evaluate their quality using as a guideline the psychometric properties of reliability, validity and clinical utility.

- Structured diagnostic interviews that provide both a dichotomous and continuous rating of PTSD symptoms are preferred.
- Synoptic frequency, intensity, and duration of a particular episode and dimensions should be assessed. It is important to determine the levels of distress as articulated by patients regarding their symptom presentation.
- Ratings of impairment and disability secondary to the symptom complex provide important information regarding the severity of the condition.
- Instruments whose reliability and validity studies contain information regarding their performance across gender, racial and ethnic groups are to be given preference, especially when the instrument is to be used with males and females of different cultures and races.
- Self-report instruments for PTSD should meet the standards for psychometric instruments established by the APA.
- When examining for the presence of traumatic events in the history of a person, the committee recommended "a set of carefully worded items that cover a range of types of events as a minimum."

Furthermore, the committee recommended that "in-depth questions need to be asked about event occurrences, perceived life threat, harm, injuries, frequency, duration, and age" (Foa, Keane, & Friedman, 2000, p. 31).

These authors have identified other important factors including: "warzone stressors, sexual assault in adulthood and childhood, robbery, accidents, technological disasters, natural disasters or hazardous exposures, sudden death of a loved one, life-threatening illness, and witnessing or experiencing violence." (Foa, Keane, & Friedman, 2000, p. 31). Finally, the committee recommended that "In evaluating stressors, carefully behaviorally-anchored terminology should be used, avoiding jargon such as abuse, rape, and so on, terms that are inherently imprecise and not universally understood in the same way and across cultures." (Foa, Keane, & Friedman, 2000, p. 31).

HEALING TRAUMA'S FALLOUT: CURRENT INFORMATION ON TREATMENTS AND CONTROVERSIES

The Controversy Over Critical Incident Stress Debriefing

Van der Kolk and McFarlane remind us that "Merely uncovering memories is not enough; they need to be modified and transformed (i.e., placed in the proper context and reconstructed in a personally meaningful way)" (p. 19).

This is important to note; too many of our students tend to think that un-covering or a simple debriefing is all that is necessary.

Van der Kolk and McFarlane continue: "Because the essence of the trauma is that it once confronted the victim with unacceptable reality, the patient needs to find a way of confronting the hidden secrets that no one, including the patient wants to face." (Van der Kolk and McFarlane in Langer, 1990). How do we proceed with this challenge?

In the 1970s, Jeffrey Mitchell, Ph.D., created a system of debriefing aimed specifically at "first responders" (fire-fighters, police, and ambulance responders) whose job constantly exposed them to potentially traumatic situations. Mitchell's work was soon assumed as the norm of response in any traumatic situation and anyone related to crisis or trauma work learned how to apply the model.

Rumblings of questions started to surface in the late 1990s, particularly with an article by Avery and Orner (1998) in *Traumatic Stress Points,* a pub-lication of the International Society for Traumatic Stress Studies. Trauma victims were treated in groups shortly after the occurrence of the trauma. The groups were clearly structured. They followed a very rigid system, which had six levels:

1. Introductory phase and ground rules of the model.
2. Factual phase, in which group members would recite their memo-ries of their experiences.
3. Emotional phase, in which group members would express their emotional experiences during the traumatic event.
4. Symptom phase, in which group members would report any un-usual experiences during the event.
5. Teaching phase, in which the group leader would give members some information about their normal and abnormal reactions after this type of experience.
6. Reentry phase—helping the group members to integrate the expe-rience and return to their normal lives. (p. 12)

The use of the model spread rapidly, beyond the initial groups to all persons who had experienced traumatic events. But at the end of the 1990s, research information started to be published that questioned not only the helpfulness of the model but, in fact, suggested that it may be responsible for more complicated traumatic reactions.

In reporting on the psychosocial aspects of 9-11 and the professional response to them, Rob Waters, writing in the *Psychotherapy Networker* (2002), tells us:

While many applauded this effort (of untold numbers of volunteers who turned up to be helpful and render "psychological first aid," in many cases applying the Mitchell model,) a group of 19 psychologists, some of them prominent trauma specialists, distributed an open letter within a week of the 9-11 attack, warning their colleagues to resist "descending on disaster scenes to offer help" (p. 52).

The letter questioned the effectiveness of postdisaster debriefings and suggested that therapists can help "by supporting the community structures that people naturally call upon in times of grief and suffering" (p. 52).

The letter cautioned "it is imperative that we refrain from the urge to intervene in ways that—however well intentioned—have the potential to make matters worse" (Waters, 2002).

The PTSD Research Quarterly fall 2001 reports the following: "Although Psychological Debriefing represents the most common form of intervention for recently traumatized people, there is little evidence supporting its continued use with individuals who experience severe trauma" (p. 61). The review identifies the core issues in early intervention that need to be addressed in resolving the debate over PTSD, and continues: "Based on available evidence, we propose that psychological first aid is an appropriate initial intervention but that it does not serve a therapeutic or preventive function" (p. 134). They go on to say, "When feasible, initial screening is required so that preventive interventions can be used for those individuals who may have difficulty in recovering on their own" (Litz, Gray, Bryant, & Adler, 2002, p. 134).

Even though there is insufficient evidence supporting its continued use, psychosocial debriefing (PD) is routinely provided immediately after exposure to potentially traumatizing events (Mitchell & Everly, 1996; Raphael, Wilson, Meldrum, & McFarlane, 1996). This state of affairs is not surprising, considering the prevalence of trauma, the demand for efficient management of the extensive individual, corporate, and societal costs associated with chronic PTSD, the financial interests of those who provide acute interventions, and the tendency for organizations and participants to perceive PD as useful (Deahl, Gillham, Thomas, Searle, & Srinivasan, 1994; Hobfoll, Spielberger, Breznitz, Figley, & Van der Kolk, 1991; Raphael, Wilson, Meldrum, & McFarlane, 1996; Wilson, Kurtz, & Robert, 2000).

They conclude that "PD has been widely advocated for routine use after major traumatic events. Given the current state of knowledge, neither one-time groups nor individual PD can be advocated as being able to prevent the subsequent development of PTSD following a traumatic event" (p. 136).

The researchers further defend their position:

> However there may be benefits to aspects of PD, particularly when employed as part of a comprehensive management program. There appears to be evidence that it is well-received intervention for most people and even though it may not prevent later psychological sequelae, it may still be useful for screening, education and supportive functions. If Psychological Debriefing is to be used, it should be provided by experienced, well-trained practitioners, that it not be mandatory, and that potential participants be properly clinically assessed. (Deahl, Bisson, MacFarlane, & Rose in Foa, Keane, & Friedman, 2002, pp. 317–319)

A recent review of eight debriefing studies, all of which met rigorous criteria for being well-controlled, revealed no evidence that debriefing reduces the risk of PTSD, depression, or anxiety; nor were there any reductions in psychiatric symptoms across studies. In addition, in two studies, one of which included long-term follow-up, some negative effects of CISD-type debriefings on PTSD and other trauma-related symptoms were reported.

Rose, Wessley, and Bisson (2000) have concluded that "Debriefing is ineffective at best, and possibly harmful." This despite the fact that they acknowledge that, "While debriefings as currently employed may be useful for low magnitude stress exposure and symptoms, or for emergency providers, the best studies recommend that for individuals with more severe exposure to trauma, and for those who are experiencing more severe reactions such as PTSD."

The question of why debriefing may produce negative results has been considered, and early hypotheses have been formulated. One theory connects negative outcomes with heightened arousal in the early posttrauma phase and long-term psychopathology (Shalev, 2001; Bryant et al., 2000). Because verbalization of the trauma in debriefing is limited, habituation to evoked distress does not occur. The result may be an increase rather than a decrease in arousal. Any such increased distress caused by debriefing may be difficult to detect in a group setting. Thus, attempting to override dissociation and avoidance in the immediate posttrauma phase with debriefing may be detrimental to some individuals, particularly those experiencing heightened arousal. Also to be considered is the observation that the boundary between debriefing and therapy is sometimes blurred (e.g., challenging thoughts), which may increase distress in some individuals (Bryant, 2000). Finally, debriefers frequently are unable to adequately assess traumatized individuals in a group setting. They may erroneously conclude that a one-time intervention will be sufficient to prevent further symptomatology.

Practice guidelines on debriefing formulated by the International Society for Traumatic Stress Studies conclude:

> There is little evidence that debriefing prevents psychopathology. The guidelines recommend that, while debriefing is often well-received, and while it may be useful to facilitate screening of those at risk, disseminate education and referral information, and improve organizational morale, debriefing (if employed) should
>
> - be conducted by experienced, well-trained practitioners
> - not be mandatory
> - utilize some clinical assessment of potential participants
> - be accompanied by clear and objective evaluation procedures. (ISTSS, 2000)

The guidelines state that while it is premature to conclude that debriefing should be discontinued altogether, "more complex interventions for those individuals at highest risk may be the best way to prevent the development of PTSD following trauma" (ISTSS, 2000).

In a response to criticism of Critical Incident Stress Debriefing, doctors Mitchell and Everly (creators of the process) point out that

> A debriefing is merely one group intervention technique within the field of crisis intervention. The seven primary components of Critical Incident Stress Management are the following:
>
> - Precrisis education and preparedness training.
> - One-on-one psychological support sessions.
> - Disaster demobilizations and deployment briefing sessions for large groups.
> - Small group brief defusing immediately after the traumatic event (20–40 minutes in length).
> - Significant-other support programs and organizational support programs (educational and crisis intervention).
> - Critical Incident Stress Debriefings, which are structured into 1–3 hour, seven-phase group discussions of a highly stressful event.
> - Follow up and referral mechanisms for further assessment and therapy. (Mitchell & Everly, 1996, p. 35)

They go on to say that

> CISDs are used to equalize the information among the group members and instruct the participants about practical steps that can assist in recovery from the traumatic experience. One of the most important functions served by the CISD process is a screening function. It facilitates identification of group members who may need additional intervention or Psychotherapy (Mitchell & Everly, 1996, p. 36).

Hypnosis

The American Psychological Association, Division of Psychological Hypnosis, provided the following definition of hypnosis in 1993:

> Hypnosis is a procedure during which a health professional or researcher suggests that a client, patient, or subject experience changes in sensations, perceptions, thoughts, or behavior. The hypnotic context is generally established by an induction procedure. Although there are many different hypnotic inductions, most include suggestions for relaxation, calmness, and well being. Instructions to imagine or think about pleasant experiences are also commonly included in hypnotic inductions. People respond to hypnosis in different ways. Some describe their experience as an altered state of consciousness. Others describe hypnosis as a normal state of focused attention, in which they feel very calm and relaxed. Regardless of how and to what degree they respond, most people describe the experience as very pleasant. Some people are very responsive to hypnotic suggestions and others are less responsive. A person's ability to experience hypnotic suggestions can be inhibited by fears and concerns arising from some common misconceptions.
>
> Contrary to some depictions of hypnosis in books, movies or on television, people who have been hypnotized do not lose control over their behavior. They typically remain aware of who they are and where they are, and unless amnesia has been specifically suggested, they usually remember what transpired during hypnosis. Hypnosis makes it easier for people to experience suggestions, but it does not force them to have these experiences.

Cognitive Behavior Therapy

In *Excerpts from Mental Health Interventions for Disasters,* a Center for PTSD fact sheet, we learn that "there are more published well-controlled studies of cognitive behavior therapy (CBT) than there are of any other PTSD treatment. CBT treatments for PTSD include the following:

- Exposure therapy, in which patients are asked to describe their traumatic experiences in detail, on a repetitive basis, in order to reduce the arousal and distress associated with their memories.
- Cognitive therapy, which focuses on helping patients identify their trauma-related negative beliefs (e.g., guilt, distrust of others) and changing them to reduce distress.
- Stress inoculation training, in which patents are taught skills for managing and reducing anxiety (breathing, muscular relaxation, self-talk)."

Cognitive behavioral therapy has been shown to be effective in overcoming anxiety or depression and modifying undesirable behaviors.

Leahy (2003) tells us that "the cognitive therapy model is based on the view that stressful states . . . are often exacerbated by biased ways of thinking. The therapist's role is to help the patient recognize his or her idiosyncratic style of thinking and modify it through the application of evidence and logic. . . . Cognitive therapists engage patients in scientific and rational thinking by asking them to examine their presuppositions."

Leahy continues:

> The cognitive therapist recognizes that rational analysis and descriptions of thought processes may not be sufficient to mediate change. Evocation of emotion, development of motivation and experiential techniques that activate new phenomenological experiences and feelings also may be essential. The patient may need to confront reality with new thought and behaviors in order to experience, on an emotional level, the existential importance of a "rational" response or simply a new way of thinking.

The therapist helps the patient examine and reevaluate the beliefs that are interfering with healing. These beliefs may include the fear that the traumatic event will reoccur. Another aspect of this approach may include an in vivo exposure such as returning to the scene where the trauma occurred. Elements of change are measured in the Subjective Units of Distress Scale (SUDS), and this ability to measure change strengthens the experience of the effectiveness of the treatment. Some aspects of cognitive behavioral therapy that are particularly appropriate for posttraumatic experiences include Exposure Therapy, wherein clients are asked to describe their traumatic experiences in detail on a repetitive basis in order to reduce the arousal and distress. Some of our readers may recognize this as an older concept called Systematic Desensitization.

Kubany, Hill, and Owens (2004) in the first controlled PTSD treatment outcome study using cognitive therapy with battered women, had results that were of great interest. They said that "Considerable research has emphasized the importance of cognitive variables as factors that contribute to the maintenance or persistence of post-traumatic stress." When negative thoughts such as "I'm worthless" occur, the researchers tell us that "Self-punishment can have deleterious effects on a person's well being, by contributing to the maintenance of Posttraumatic Stress and depression" (p. 81).

They also quote Kubany and Wilson (2002):

> An important reason why memories of trauma do not lose their capacity to evoke emotional pain may be due to the higher order language conditioning whereby words that have acquired the ability to evoke negative

affect ("stupid—I should never have, etc.") function in effect as unconditioned stimuli in pairing with images of trauma. Evaluative self-talk narratives which accompany memories of trauma may provide thousands of reconditioning trials that effectively interfere with the natural process of emotional extinction.

The findings were that the process is not only helpful in general but, as well, it was found to be "efficacious across ethnic backgrounds," an interesting and hopeful new approach to healing this population (p. 81).

Acute Interventions After Disaster

By this time, most of us have an awareness of the importance and application of immediate crisis intervention. Shalev (2001) adds, "Several factors make the treatment of survivors, in the acute aftermath of traumatic events, extremely difficult to describe and discuss." Because the obvious aspects of need appear most urgent, the potential for psychopathology may not be recognized. However, as Shalev points out, "Secondary stressors may still be operating, expressions of distress are volatile and highly reactive to external realities." He reminds us of what Carl Rogers used to teach us at La Jolla, namely, to "trust the process." This translates to remembering that "normal healing processes are already operating, and significant assistance is provided by natural supporters and healers (e.g., relatives, community leaders) and should not be interfered with" (Shalev, 2001, p. 8).

There are times, as Shalev reminds us, when we cannot trust a system under duress and we must seek out alternatives. "An alternative model may be considered, which favors knowledge of pathogenic processes over symptom recognition" (2001). Essentially, Shalev's very important message is that there is a need for flexibility in our intervention styles.

Ruzek and Garay (1996) suggest: "In the acute aftermath of a disaster, initial interventions may be primarily practical and simple, depending on the need of those in crisis." They continue, "Some of the most pragmatic and useful interventions are those of linking survivors to community resources for food, shelter, clothing and other forms of disaster relief. Initial psychological crisis intervention may involve stabilizing and preventing an escalation of the initial crisis reactions and symptomatology."

They make another important contribution by reminding us that, "Providing psychoeducational interventions regarding typical posttraumatic reactions may serve to normalize and reduce distress for some individuals. Providing support for the mobilization of coping strategies is a key intervention." In addition, they say, "Another central task is the identification of reactions that pose a danger to self or others, or are indicative of a much greater difficulty in coping (e.g., severe acute stress disorder symptoms such as amnesia, depersonalization, and alterations in state of consciousness)." Ruzek also reminds us that in the past, when patients came to hospitals for physical injuries, there was little concern about their psychological or emotional needs. "In many cases psychological trauma has been shown to be related to physical trauma. Of late a greater awareness of this schism has developed" (Ruzek, 1996).

Although these concepts are of great value, reality does not always support them. This awareness of the need for sensitive intervention, while not mandatory, can only be achieved with the appropriate training of staff.

Helpful responses cannot be structured or rigidly imposed. Every level of staff involved in working with these patients must be made aware of these issues.

The optimal time for these interventions is unclear. On one hand, the very early days that follow traumatic events may constitute a critical or sensitive period, during which neuronal plasticity is enhanced (Shalev et al., 1992), and indelible aversive learning occurs (Shalev, Rogel-Fuchs, & Pitman, 1992). On the other hand, most trauma survivors do not present to treatment before having endured weeks of suffering, possibly because they, and others around them, see the initial distress and the associated symptoms as a normal response.

An interesting model develped by Foa, Hearst-Ikeda, and Perry (1963) was created to meet patients' needs. This included, "A range of psychological interventions may be appropriately applied with this population, including psychoeducation about medical procedures and trauma and stress reactions, training in stress-management, medication, and exposure treatments."

In addition, they suggest that "early interventions may help prevent development of PTSD among some trauma survivors." Foa, Hearst-Ikeda, and Perry (1963), for example,

> delivered 4 sessions of cognitive-behavioral therapy education, Breathing/relaxation, Imaginal and in vivo exposure, and Cognitive restructuring—to recent female victims of sexual and nonsexual assault. Referral sources in this study included hospital emergency room personnel. Subjects were assessed within 3 weeks of the assault and treatment was started immediately following assessment. Five months post-assault, individuals who received this early post-trauma care were significantly less depressed and experienced fewer re-experiencing symptoms than a matched control group. None of the treated group showed depression or more than six PTSD symptoms; 56% of the control group reported

moderate-to-severe depression and 33% had more than six PTSD symptoms. This study provided evidence that a brief cognitive-behavioral program administered shortly after an assault can accelerate rate of improvement of trauma-related psychological problems."

Doing follow ups and outreach with medical patients to check for post-trauma problems experienced after hospital discharge was also suggested. Families of deceased patients, who are now secondary victims of the trauma, must be attended to as well. These families may develop a range of psychological problems and can benefit from support and counseling.

COMPASSION FATIGUE

All of us who work with traumatized populations must be aware of this phenomenon. Originally created by Dr. Charles Figley, it is not identical to burnout, as some may think. Figley (1995) says,

> In contrast to burnout which emerges gradually and is a result of emotional exhaustion, (compassion fatigue) can emerge suddenly with little warning. In addition to a more rapid onset of symptoms, in contrast to burnout, there is a sense of helplessness and confusion, and a sense of isolation from supporters; the symptoms are often disconnected from real causes, and yet there is faster recovery rate (p. 12).

David Baldwin (1995, May 19) summarizes it thus: "An additional aspect of traumatic exposure affects primarily the workers who help trauma and disaster victims. These people include psychologists and other mental health workers, exposed to an overdose of victim suffering."
Baldwin continues,

> Professions who are involved in working with trauma such as emergency workers, physicians, fire, police, search and rescue, psychologists etc. are at risk for secondary traumatization (also known as compassion fatigue). . . . The symptoms here are usually less severe than PTSD-like symptoms experienced by direct victims in a disaster.

However, Baldwin (1995, May 19) points out that

> they can affect the livelihoods and careers of those with considerable training and experience working with disaster and trauma survivors. . . . As you might expect the risk increases when traumatic exposures are unexpected or among those without adequate preparation.

He lists three risk factors:

1. Exposure to the stories or images of multiple disaster victims.
2. Your empathic sensitivity to their suffering.
3. Any unresolved emotional issues that relate affectively symbolically to the suffering seen.

CARE FOR THE CAREGIVERS

Imagine yourself working in a situation in which, throughout the day, you are confronted with people no different than you or your loved ones, but whose lives are threatened by sudden unexpected events. Take a moment and visualize yourself in this situation. Tune in to your body as well as your mind as you do this little exercise. How long do you think you can maintain your sensitivity, caring, and objectivity if you are constantly confronted with "mass death, deaths of children, grotesque injury, and severe human-caused injury. Such exposure may exact a powerful emotional toll which is too often accepted as 'just part of the job' and ignored by program administrators and Trauma Center staff themselves" (Ruzek & Garay, 1996).

Ruzek and others remind us that trauma workers and clinicians who provide trauma services in a disaster "may themselves become overwhelmed by caring for the acute survivors or by the effects of the trauma that they have suffered directly." These groups, including medical, nursing, mental health and ambulance personnel, and others of this ilk must "recognize their own vulnerability to the same reactions as those they are treating" (Ruzek & Garay, 1996).

We must be sensitive to the needs of these workers and provide interventions for their acute care during and after disasters, if necessary. It is quite clear to those of us who have experience in situations like these, that we are only human, and, thus, quite vulnerable. Being exposed to painful experiences like trauma can have a difficult effect on us, and all of us in the helping professions need to stay in touch with our own physical and psychological needs as we work to help others. If we fail to do this we may be failing our patients as well as ourselves. In the case of mass traumas, there is a strong possibility that we have been confronting the same experiences as our patients. In working with individual trauma we may very easily identify with our patients' experiences. We may, in fact, have experienced situations similar to those that patients report. We must be sensitive to our own vulnerabilities and monitor ourselves for the possibilities of our own symptoms, while at the same time maintaining our boundaries.

PREVENTIVE INTERVENTIONS

Having reviewed the more productive and less productive approaches to trauma intervention, we now need to look at "preventive interventions." The goal of preventive intervention is to find a medium or media that professionals can use to help the trauma patient in the immediate aftermath of the experience in a manner that will not only prevent the development of PTSD but as will create or increase resilience.

One snowy day, I was driving along a road in Vermont when I saw that a car and a pickup truck were aligned on the same side of the road, facing each other. An accident had apparently just occurred. Getting out of my car, I saw that a family with a child were all in their car crying, very upset. There were, however, many people with them, all reporting that the ambulance had been called and assuring me that the injuries were not very severe. As I looked up, I saw two young men leaning against their pickup truck, which had skidded over from the northbound lane to the southbound lane. There it had hit the oncoming car, and hence, it was stopped on the wrong side of the road. They were driving in the direction away from the ski hills and had skis on their truck. I assumed that they were on their way home from a full day on the ski hills.

It appeared that they had skidded, lost control of their car, and ended up in the oncoming lane, causing this accident. I went over and talked to them about what had happened. They had indeed been returning from a ski outing when their car landed in the oncoming lane. I listened to their description of the accident and just said a few understanding words. Quite unexpectedly, one of them, a huge sturdy young man, suddenly threw his arms around me and hugged me and started to cry. He told me that he was driving home from a day on the slopes, when the road suddenly became very slippery and his car had skidded into the other lane, causing the accident. He talked and talked, and I was as reassuring and supportive as I could be (in what I was later to process as "preventive debriefing"). It was clear to me that the two young men in the truck were the forgotten victims. They, too, needed support and debriefing as much as the more obvious victims of the crash. In situations like this one, we need to take stock of our own focus and make sure it as broad as possible so that we can survey and recognize all of the players. Sometimes the quiet, withdrawn person off in a corner is in greater pain than the more histrionic one that all can see. We need to acknowledge the needs of all of them in a preventive manner.

Welzant and Lowenstein (2001) report that "In medical settings, a consultation-liaison outreach model has been advocated for addressing the psychiatric needs of injured disaster survivors. The identification of high-risk groups is one task of disaster mental health personnel."

Other such groups include "The elderly, those with predisaster psychiatric conditions, and the acutely bereaved have been identified as being at highest risk for psychiatric sequelae following a disaster. . . . Those with high levels of exposure and responsibility for responding to the traumatic event may also be at high risk" (Welzant & Lowenstein, 2001, p. 5).

Hospital personnel have become aware of the contributions that they can make to preventive intervention in trauma situations. "Psychological triage is a major task of disaster mental health work. Those who are in need of more than crisis intervention services are referred for ongoing mental health treatment" (Ruzek, 1996). Although we often fail to recognize it, "In a disaster, however, the usual referral resources may be compromised by the disaster itself, or may be overwhelmed by the volume of requests for services, slowing the usual referral process considerably" (Ruzek & Garay, 1996). It is essential therefore that mental health agencies create emergency and contingency plans.

OTHER RESOURCES

I have always found, both from my own experience and that of my clients, that writing is an extremely valuable medium for healing. I encourage people to keep journals. These allow them to express their feelings as they move through the changes in their lives. In addition, it allows them to visibly acknowledge the changes that occur as they keep track of them. Clients often come in to tell me that they reread older journals and were astounded at the changes that they saw in themselves. This has an extremely powerful reinforcement for them and allows them to respect their healing, the change experience and their growth. Often they will use varied modalities such as poetry or drama to express themselves, all of which are very helpful.

The American Psychological Association (2003) has issued the following material on this topic:

> Writing about difficult, even traumatic, experiences appears to be good for health on several levels, raising immunity and other health measures and improving life functioning. . . . Deep disclosure improves mood, objective and subjective health, and the ability to function well. Classic studies by psychologist James W. Pennebaker, PhD and his colleagues have proved the health value of personal disclosure. In a class of 50 healthy undergraduates were assigned to write about either traumatic experiences or superficial topics for four days in a row. Six weeks after the writing sessions, students in the trauma group reported more positive moods and fewer illnesses than those writing about everyday experiences. Furthermore, improved measures of cellular immune-system function and fewer visits to the student health center for those writing about painful experiences suggested that confronting traumatic experiences was physically beneficial. (Pennebaker, Kiecolt-Glaser, & Glaser, 1988, p. 241)

At the Dallas Memorial Center for Holocaust Studies, Pennebaker and colleagues did a physiological assessment while videotaping interviews of more than 60 Holocaust survivors. They "classified each survivor, based on the interview, as a low, midlevel, or high 'discloser.' High and midlevel disclosers were significantly healthier a year after the interviews than the 'low disclosers'" (1988, p. 243).

In 1999, Joshua Smyth and Arthur Stone and colleagues at the State University of New York (SUNY) at Stony Brook assigned patients with asthma and rheumatoid arthritis either to write about the most stressful event of their lives or to write about a neutral topic. Four months later, asthma patients in the experimental group showed improvements in lung function and arthritis patients in the experimental group showed a reduction in disease severity. In all, 47% of the patients who disclosed stressful events showed clinically relevant improvement, whereas only 24% of the control group exhibited such improvement.

This chapter raises our awareness of some of the greatest emotional, mental, and even physical pain that humans can experience. Tragically, much of this pain is created by other humans. While we need to focus much of our attention on developing more helpful ways of healing each other, equal amounts of our energies should be directed toward ways of altering human behavior, in the hopes of preventing the horrors and nightmares that we have, sadly, learned to inflict upon each other.

REFERENCES

Avery, A., & Orner, R. (1998). First report of psychological debriefing abandoned: The end of an era? *Traumatic Stress Points, 12,* 3–4.

Baldwin, D. (1995, May 19). *David Baldwin's trauma pages.* Retrieved from www.trauma-pages.com

Bryant, R. A., Harvey, A. G., Dang, S. T., Sackville, T., & Basten, C. (2000). "Cognitive therapy." In *Excerpts from mental health interventions for disasters: A National Center for PTSD fact sheet.*

Cloitrer, M. (1998). In Folette, V. M., "Cognitive therapy." In *Excerpts from mental health interventions for disasters: A National Center for PTSD fact sheet* (p. 278).

Deahl, M., Bisson, J. I., MacFarlane, A., & Rose, S. (2000). Effective treatments for PTSD: Practice guidelines. In E. B. Foa, T. M. Keane, & M. J. Friedman, (2002), *International Society for Traumatic Stress Studies* (pp. 317–319).

Deahl, M., Gillham, A., Thomas, J., Searle, M., & Srinivasan, M. (1994). Psychological sequelae following the Gulf War: Factors associated with subsequent morbidity and the effectiveness of psychological debriefing. *British Journal of Psychiatry, 165,* 60–65.

Deering, C. G., Glover, S. G., Ready, D., & Eddleman, H. C. (2002, June). The effect of loss and trauma on substance use behavior. *Alarcon.*

Executive Committee of the American Psychological Association Division of Psychological Hypnosis. (1993, fall). *Psychological Hypnosis: A Bulletin of Division 30,* pp. 2, 7.

Figley, C. R., (1995). *Compassion fatigue* (p. 12). New York: Brunner/Mazel.

Foa, E. B., Hearst-Ikeda, D., & Perry, K. J. (1963). Evaluation of a brief cognitive-behavioral program for the prevention of chronic PTSD in recent assault victims. *Journal of Consulting and Clinical Psychology, 63,* 48–955.

Foa, E. B., Keane, T. M., & Friedman, M. J. (2000). *Effective treatments for PTSD* (p. 31). New York: Guilford Press.

Folette, V. M. (1998). *Knowing and not knowing about trauma implications for therapy.* University of Oregon.

Gaensbauer, T. J., & Siegel, C. H. (1995). Therapeutic approaches to posttraumatic stress. *Infant Mental Health Journal, 16,* 292–305.

Gurvits, T. G., Shenton, M. R., Hokama, H., Ohta, H., Lasko, N. B., Gilberson, M. W., et al. (1996). Magnetic resonance imaging study of hippocampal volume in chronic combat-related post traumatic stress disorder. *Biol Psychiatry, 40,* 192–199.

Herman, J. L. (1992). *Trauma and recovery.* New York: Basic Books.

Hobfoil, Spielberger, Figley, & van der Kolk. (1991). Early intervention for trauma: Current status and future. In U.S. Department of Veteran's Affairs, National Center for PTSD fact sheet titled *Early interventions for trauma: Current status and future directions.* Retrieved July 13, 2000 online.

Hobfoll, S. E., Spielberger, C. D., Breznitz, S., Figley, C., Folkman, S., Green, B. L., et al. (1991). War-related stress: Addressing the stress of war and other traumatic events. *American Psychologist, 46,* 848–855.

ISTSS. (2004). 20th Annual Meeting.

Kessler, R. C., Sonnega, A., Bromet, E., Hughes, M., & Nelson, C. B. (1995). PTSD information for women's health providers. National Center for PTSD, reported in Ozer & Weiss (2004).

Kubany, E. S., Hill, E. E., Owens, J. A., Iannce-Spencer, C., McCaig, M. A., Tremayne, K. J., et al. (2004). Cognitive trauma therapy for battered women with PTSD. *Journal of Consulting & Clinical Psychology, 72*(1), 3–18.

Kubany, E. S., & Watson, E. B. (2002). Cognitive trauma therapy for formerly battered women with PTSD. Quoted in E. S. Kubany, E. E. Hill, & J. A. Owens (2003). Cognitive trauma therapy for Battered women with PTSD. *Journal of Traumatic Stress, 16*(2), 81–91.

Kulka, R. A., Schlenger, W. E., Fairbank, J. A., Hough, R. L., Jordan, B. K., Marmar, C. R., et al. (1990). *Trauma and the Vietnam War generation: Report of findings from the National Vietnam Veterans Readjustment Study* (pp. 503–520). New York: Brunner/Mazel.

Leahy, R. L., & Holland, S. J. (2000). Post traumatic stress disorder. In R. L. Leahy

& S. J. Holland, *Treatment plans and interventions for depression and anxiety disorders*. New York: Guilford Publishing.

Litz, B. T., Gray, M. J., Bryant, R. A., & Adler, A. B. (2002). Early intervention for trauma: Current status and future directions. *Clinical Psychology, 9*(2), 112–134.

Mitchell, J. T., & Everly, Jr., G. S. (1996). *Critical incident stress debriefing (CISD): An operations manual for the prevention of traumatic stress among emergency services and disaster workers*. Ellicott City, MD: Chevron.

Pennebaker, J. W. (1999). The effects of traumatic disclosure on physical and mental health: The value of writing and talking about upsetting events. *International Journal of Emergency Mental Health, 1*(1), 9–18.

Pennebaker, J. W., Kiecolt-Glaser, J. K., & Glaser, R. (1988). Disclosure of traumas and immune function: Health implications for psychotherapy. *Journal of Consulting and Clinical Psychology, 56*, 239–245.

Raphael, B., Wilson, J., Meldrum, L., & McFarlane, A. C. (1996). First report of psychological debriefing abandoned—the end of an era? In A. Avery, S. King, & R. Orner (1999), *Traumatic Stress Points, 12*(3).

Raphael, B., & Wilson, J. P. (Eds.). (2000). *Psychological debriefing: Theory, practice and evidence*. New York: Cambridge University Press.

Rose, S., Wessley, & Bisson, J. I. (2000). *Mental health intervention for disasters. A National center for PTSD fact sheet*.

Ruzek, J. I., & Garay, K. (1996). Hospital trauma care and management of trauma-related psychological problems. *NCP Clinical Quarterly, 6*(4).

Shalev, A. Y. (2001). "What is post-traumatic stress disorder?" *Journal Of Clinical Psychiatry, 62*(Suppl. 17), 4–10.

Shalev, A. Y., Rogel-Fuchs, Y., & Pitman, R. K. (1992). Conditioned fear and psychological trauma. *Biological Psychiatry, 31*, 863–856.

Smyth, J. M., Stone, A. A., Hurewitz, A., & Kaell, A. (1999). Effects of writing about stressful experiences on symptom reduction in patients with asthma or rheumatoid arthritis. *Journal of the American Medical Association, 281*, 1304–1309.

Teicher, M. (2000). Wounds that time won't heal. *Cerebrum, 2*(4), 50–67.

Tutu, D. (2006, January 29). *An interview with Archbishop Desmond Tutu*. All Things Considered.

Van der Kolk, B. A., McFarlane, A. C., & Weisaeth, L. (Eds.). (1996). *Traumatic stress: The effects of overwhelming experience on mind, body and society* (p. 19). New York: Guilford Press.

Van der Kolk, B., & McFarlane, A. (1989). In E. J. Langer, *Mindfulness*. Reading, MA: Addison-Wesley.

Waters, R. (2002). *Psychotherapy Networker, 54*.

Weiss, D. S., Marmar, C. R., Schlenger, W. E., Fairbank, J. A., Jordan, B. K., Hough, R. L., et al. (1992). The prevalence of lifetime and partial post-traumatic stress disorder in Vietnam theater veterans. *Journal of Traumatic Stress, 5*, 365–376.

Welzant, V., & Loewenstein, J. (2001). Psychiatry and the aftermath of September 11, 2001. *American Journal of Psychiatry, 28*(2), 1, 4–6.

Wilson, J. P., Kurtz, & Robert, R. (2000). Assessing PTSD in couples and partners: The dyadic dance of trauma. *National Center for PTSD Clinical Quarterly, 9*(3).

CHAPTER 8

Trauma and the Body

The body remembers.

> —Babette Rothschild (2000)

The body keeps the score.

> —Bessell Van der Kolk (2004)

Knowledge was so important to the development of civilization that it seemed justifiable to deny the body's claim to equality. We are witnessing a new respect for the body and are moving away from the old dichotomy that saw mind and body as two separate and distinct entities.

> — Alexander Lowen (1976)

FIRST DO NO HARM:
CREATING A SAFE PLACE

One of the most important things we can do with traumatized people is to teach them how to create their own "safe place" before they start to approach the intense pain of the trauma. In my earlier book (with Bloch, 1998), we said,

> The concept of a safe place is key to all of our work. . . . Loss of safety is key to the crisis-trauma experience. In reality the very place that can help the individual feel safe may have been destroyed, either concretely or emotionally. In natural disasters the very home the person lives in may have been destroyed. In an interpersonal breakdown the person the client counted on for support, love and emotional security may either be sick, injured or dying, or may have decided to leave the relationship. Loss of safety is one of the most significant experiences of crisis and trauma.

A safe place can be created in a number of different modalities. The most obvious safe place is, first and foremost in the relationship with the therapist. This has to be a sacred trust. Many traumatized people are so distrustful that even the slightest change in schedule can be a cause for their distrust (p. 174).

In their interesting workbook for clients, *Life After Trauma: A Workbook For Healing,* Rosenbloom and Williams identify five core psychological needs: safety, trust, control, self-esteem, and intimacy. These needs should be kept in mind in all of your work with clients, but particularly when you move into the sphere of bodywork.

THE BODY REMEMBERS

Babette Rothschild, in her valuable book *The Body Remembers* (2000) teaches us that "trauma is a psychophysical experience, even when the traumatic event causes no bodily harm. That traumatic events exact a toll on the body as well as on the mind is a well-documented and agreed-on conclusion of the psychiatric community as attested to in the DSM IV" (p. 6).

She goes on to say that "despite a plethora of study and writing on the neurobiology and psychobiology of stress, trauma and PTSD, the psychotherapist has until now had few tools for healing the traumatized body as well as the traumatized mind" (p. 5). In addition, Rothchild notes, "trauma continues to intrude with visual, auditory and/or other somatic reality on the lives of its victims" (p. 6).

Several years ago, I was driving a friend to her destination in a rural section of Vermont. We were driving on a picturesque country road that had one curve after another. I noticed that she had left an uncovered cup of hot tea on the window ledge and mentioned it to her. Since she did not respond, and since I knew how curvy the terrain was, I automatically reached over to put the cup into a safer place. In doing this, despite my knowledge of the road, I missed a turn and found myself and my car abruptly and painfully halted. I had, unfortunately, missed one of those many turns and had hit a tree head on. Since I was sitting somewhat closer to the wheel than others might, my airbag exploded, hitting my face and head directly. The only thing I remembered right after that was lying on the floor between the two front seats as well–meaning passersby tried to help us. They tried to pull me out but were unsuccessful. Eventually, the local ambulance brigade arrived and took both of us to the emergency room of the nearest hospital. There I waited until I could be completely examined. The first thing that happened was that my face became embroidered with tens of stitches as a result of the impact of the airbag on my eyeglasses, but the worst was yet to come. When they asked me to raise my left arm, I found that that was impossible, as my seat belt had gotten under my arm and pulled at it mercilessly. When they asked me to stand up and walk into an x-ray room, I discovered that my balance was nonexistent. This was a rather terrifying situation. I was seriously afraid that I would not be able to reconnect with my balance system. It took several months before this part of my brain remembered what it was supposed to do, and my husband vividly remembers that I lost all of my confidence in cars for quite a while. Not only would I not drive as I had for nearly 30 years, but I could not sit in the front seat when someone else was driving. Gradually, I started to drive again, but for a long time I was unable to drive on that particular stretch of winding roads. The most emotionally painful aspect of the impact was, however, the flashbacks that it created. These flashbacks took me to the single most painful experience of my life. A week before my ninth birthday, I watched helplessly as my brave older brother, while sleigh riding on a hill in the park, lost control of his sled. The sled hit a tree with him on board, and 14 hours later I was told that he had died. As I hit that tree on the charming little Vermont road, the last thing I remembered before blacking out was something inside of me whispering, "Oh, now it's my turn!" The assumption of potential death, particularly involving a tree, had obviously been waiting in my subconscious all of those years. Without consciously having been aware of it, it had been stored someplace within my psyche ever since his death. Seeing that tree now looming over my car in all of its power, so similar to the one that had killed my brother, created a flashback that my psyche had been wrestling with ever since his death. At that moment, and for months afterward, my body's violation produced flashbacks to the most painful day of my childhood, and, indeed, my life. Even today, as I drive past that area, my body clenches up and reminds me that it was a place of terror and trauma, a place where I thought I was surely going to meet death in almost exactly the way that my brother did.

Research done by Van der Kolk has shown that "the imprint of therapy doesn't 'sit' in the verbal, understanding part of the brain, . . . People process their trauma from the bottom up—body to mind—not top down." He goes on to tell us, "To do effective therapy we need to do things that change the way people regulate these core functions, which probably can't be done by words . . . alone" (2004, p. 35).

In my book (with Bloch) (Wainrib, in Wainrib & Bloch, 1998), I described a series of body exercises that I had developed over the years of working with patients who were experiencing life crises or trauma. I will re-peat some of them in this chapter as well as describe other more recent and more related work.

THE BODY AS A SAFE PLACE

In the 1970s, a patient was referred to me who had just arrived from another city. After several sessions, she told me that she really felt that working with me was very helpful, but that the one component that was missing was bodywork. I took her comment seriously and subsequently went to New York and Connecticut to train with Dr. Arne Welhaven, Dr. John Pierrakos, and Dr. Alexander Lowen, all leaders in the emerging Bioenegetics move-ment, an approach that used the body to heal the mind. I found their work fascinating and of special help for people who had the tendency to intellec-tualize and rationalize (and often not really get much better). At that time, we talked primarily about life crises, since the concept of trauma was not yet generally recognized.

After I became involved with crisis and trauma patients, I realized how helpful bodywork could be. This was, of course, before Van der Kolk and others subscribed to it fully, but it was, nevertheless, a positive move for my own work. However, for a considerable amount of time, I have been ori-ented to therapeutic work that incorporates both the mind and the body.

Many years later, Rothschild (2000, p. 100) tells us, "The potential benefits of being able to use the body as a resource in the treatment of trauma and PTSD, regardless of the treatment model, cannot be overem-phasized." After our experience with bodywork, it is not surprising that Rothschild adds, "Employing the client's own awareness of the state of the body—his perception of the precise, coexisting sensations that arise from external and internal stimuli—is a most practical tool in the treatment of trauma" (p. 100).

In addition, Van der Kolk (2004) comments on this subject: "Funda-mentally, words can't integrate the disorganized sensations and action patterns that form the core of the trauma; treatment needs to integrate the sensations and actions that have become 'stuck.'" Many of us who have worked in this milieu will, I am sure, recognize this phenomenon. Van der Kolk describes his experience: "I saw very vividly how important it is for people to overcome their sense of helplessness after a trauma by actively doing something. Preventing people from doing things after a trauma, that's one of the things that makes trauma a trauma" (p. 35).

We need to help our patients to reconnect with their bodies in our work as a means of freeing them from their traumatic experiences.

SUCCESSFUL EXERCISES

What follows are a variety of exercises that I have developed and used successfully for many years, with hundreds of patients. They include parts of various methods, including visual imagery, self-hypnosis, and others. Although some of these exercises are based on exercises in my previous book, certain changes were developed more recently. I have found them to be of great value because they give the client a skill that can be used either when working on painful memories with the therapist or when they feel that the horrors are about to resurface anywhere. I have used them to train professionals as well as patients. Teaching portable skills such as the ones we are about to describe can be of great help. They give the client an anchor that is always available to her.

Other exercises are an outgrowth of work done in relaxation and stress reduction. When using the exercises, be aware of the differing needs of the "constricted" and the "dilated" client. The constricted client may be very resistant to affective expression. Yet this is the person who may most benefit from them. The dilated client may be anxious to move into a more dramatic affective expression, but your role here is to direct the energies toward successful focusing on problem solving, and further dilating the client's affective function.

Remember also how vulnerable a traumatized individual is. They may easily abdicate their power to you and allow you to lead them into exercises that would ordinarily be unacceptable to them. The helper needs to use good judgment in deciding the relevant effectiveness of the exercise with any client. The client's own self-respect should never be compromised. One way to overcome this is to have the helper do the exercise along with the client. This helps to overcome the client's resistance and feelings of discomfort. This is especially true for highly defended, intellectualized clients. One such client told me that she would have to question my qualifications as a therapist if I had to resort to nonverbal exercises. Much later, when she was terminating her therapy and reviewing what she had learned and what was effective, she confided that the work she had done in the nonverbal mode, after her initial resistance was overcome, was the most powerful and unforgettable of her therapy. These can be potentially powerful tools, but they must be used in an atmosphere of significant respect for the client. As well, it cannot be overstressed that it is really important for the helper to be comfortable in doing these exercises. If the helper feels uncomfortable, that discomfort will be experienced by the client. In addition, the client has been through a difficult time and does not want to appear as a performing monkey to himself or to the helper.

Progressive Relaxation

This is the most basic exercise. Directions for a typical progressive relaxation exercise are as follows: Lie down in a comfortable place. Breathe easily and regularly. Focus on your breathing. As you inhale, feel your breath bring peace and calm to every part of your body. Do this for a few minutes. At your next inhalation, point your toes and stretch the bottoms of your feet. Hold your breath, and as you do so, hold your feet in the outstretched position. Then gently exhale and relax your feet.

Breathe comfortably for a few minutes. At your next inhalation, tighten your leg muscles and stretch your legs. Hold this position as you hold your breath, then gently exhale and relax your legs.

Breathe comfortably for a few minutes. Feel your legs becoming warm, heavy, and relaxed. When you next inhale, tighten the muscles of your buttocks; hold this tightness as you hold your breath. Gently exhale and relax your buttocks.

Breathe comfortably for a few minutes, then inhale and tighten your stomach muscles; hold this tightness as you hold your breath. Gently exhale and relax.

Feel the whole lower half of your body becoming heavy, warm, and relaxed. Inhale and make your hands into two fists and pull your arms straight down, as if you were pulling them out of their sockets. Hold your breath and hold your hands and arms in this tight position, then gently exhale and relax your arms and hands.

Breathe comfortably for a few minutes, then inhale and pull your head down and touch your chest with your chin. Hold this position as you hold your breath for as long as you can.

Breathe comfortably for a few minutes, then exhale and relax your head and your chest muscles. Now your whole body is feeling warm, heavy, and relaxed.

Breathe comfortably for a few minutes, and when you next inhale, raise your shoulders up to your ears and hold them there as you hold your breath for as long as you can. Then exhale and relax your head and neck.

Breathe comfortably for a few minutes, then inhale and scrunch your face up and tighten all of your facial muscles. Become aware of how much tension you are carrying on your face and tighten all of those areas. Hold this position as you hold your breath for as long as you can, and as you exhale, relax your face muscles and feel all of the tightness dissolve.

Now breathe comfortably for a while. If there is any part of your body that still feels tense, visualize your breath as a ray of soft warmth that can be directed to that tight place to relax it and heal it. Stay in this position for as long as you wish.

Think of a code word, such as "peace" or "calm" for the way you feel when you are relaxed, so that you can return to this position any time you need to. Practice saying your code word and feeling your whole body relaxed, warm, and heavy as it is now.

Creating a Safe Place

The first part of the exercise is a traditional self-hypnosis technique. It can be done after the exercise above or on its own. Teach the client to visualize herself walking down a flight of stairs. There are 20 steps in the staircase, and she will count them as she or he walks down. The usual process is to slowly count backward from 20 to one speaking at all times in a soothing, peaceful voice.

When the client gets to the bottom step, the therapist will direct her to visualize a place that she may either know of in reality or which she has imagined. The essence of this place is that it feels completely secure to her and has no possible associations to anything threatening. The concept of the complete safety of the place must be reinforced, and if the client feels that she has never actually experienced any place in which she felt totally secure, ask her to imagine what that would feel like. She can subsequently create that image in her mind.

After she has found and identified this place, reinforce a sense of safety by telling her to visualize herself more fully protecting this location by covering it with an invisible dome. This dome will allow her to see anything she wants to outside of it but prevent any person outside of the dome to see anything within it.

In other words, she is invisible to anything in the outside world, completely protected in this comfortable, entirely safe environment. Emphasize to the client that this place is totally invisible to anyone except herself, and that in it she can feel safe, relaxed and comfortable, maintaining the sense of relaxation which she has developed on her way down the stairs.

As you practice doing this exercise with clients, get in touch with your own "safe place." Find some place in your life where you can feel invisible and protected, and get in touch with the significant security that this image can create.

After the safe place has been created and the client has experienced being there for a little while, give her some kind of small object that she can hold in her hand. I use stones from my brook that I polish specifically for this purpose.

Have the client hold the stone in her hand comfortably, but tightly, as she continues to lie down with her eyes closed, focusing on the comfort and safety of the safe place. Then, direct her to become aware of the peace, tranquility, and security that she experiences in her body at this time. After she has done this, have her maintain that quality of peace and safety by envisaging this sense of comfort flowing into the stone. Having the stone retain the feelings creates the suggestion that they can always be accessed. In this manner, simply holding the stone will enable her to come back to this safe place at any time or in any place that she feels that it can be of help.

Some of my traumatized clients never travel without their stone and their safe place. One client carried her stone down the aisle as she got married. Others have carried it to distant places.

In our previous book (1998), we said "The most important piece of this visualization . . . is the security of the client. The client must chose to take into the safe place any of the icons or objects of personal security, whether concrete or abstract" (p. 174).

Breathing

Essential to all attempts to help an individual achieve a sense of calm is the use of the most powerful tool within each of us: our breathing. If the person can become aware of how effective the use of breathing is, the ability to change the stress level is always available. Any of these exercises can be done standing up or lying down.

Breathe comfortably and easily and imagine your breath as a healing presence that enters your body to bring it peace. Direct your breath to a place below your navel, which in yoga is called the *Hara.* Imagine your breath going down to that place and calming all of the body as it does this. Then become aware of any part of your body that is tense. Bring your breath to that muscle or area and become aware of how much more relaxed it can become as your breath touches it. Now place your hand on the spot below your abdomen where you are directing your breath. Feel your arm becoming more and more relaxed as you do this. Continue for as long as you need to feel your body relaxing.

CHOOSING LIFE EXERCISES

In our chapter on spirituality, we make reference to the fact that many people live in great pain, and that some people's pain is so great that they struggle daily with the decision to chose life. The following are exercises developed to strengthen the resolve to choose life, an experience that sometimes can only flicker vaguely when a person has been through a traumatic situation.

Although Jennifer Louden published this exercise in a book called *The Woman's Comfort Book* (1992), I give all of our male readers permission and encouragement to use the exercise as well.

Choose Life

Here are Louden's (1992) directions:

> Pick a time when you can be alone. Close your eyes and relax. Focus on your breathing. If you Value your breathing, you are choosing life. Realize that each breath you take is irreplaceable, a one time only event. Breathe in and out a few times and let this fact sink in. Now hold your hands. With your eyes still closed caress and explore your hands. Absorb the fact that this is the only pair of hands like these in the universe. Nowhere else does this pair of hands exist. Let your hands touch your opposite wrists and forearms. Stroke your skin and muscle. Allow your hands to travel up to your biceps and shoulders. Breathing deeply, hug yourself. Focus on your breath again. Like your breath, each moment in your life is unique and precious. Say to yourself or aloud "I grant myself the right to exist and flourish" (p. 49).

Here I Am

This is a seemingly simple yet very powerful and empowering exercise. It needs to be done in an environment of quiet and peace, so that the client can focus completely.

Have the client stand up, with face turned upward, facing the sky, but with eyes closed. Instruct him to extend his arms outward in front of him, with palms facing upward. Allow him to spend a few minutes breathing comfortably in this position. When he feels comfortable with this part of the experience, tell him to inhale deeply, and as he exhales, to say (or, if this is uncomfortable for him, to think to himself) the simple words: "Here I am." After he has said (or thought) these words, allow him a few minutes to continue the deep breathing and then to repeat them.

This should be done several times. Frequently, the client will demonstrate some strong affect, and at this time, it is good to start the processing. Allow the client to free associate about the feelings or associations he has experienced, as well as about whatever experiences they may conjure up. These may be experiences related to the traumatic event, either spiritual or otherwise. As well, they may bring back earlier memories, some related to the traumatic experience and others related to more protected situations. Help him to understand the connection between this exercise, his experience of trauma, the somewhat forgotten strengths, and the potential he may have for becoming empowered in dealing with the experience.

OTHER HEALING AND AFFIRMING EXERCISES

The following excerpt is reproduced from my 1998 book because my students found it to be extremely valuable. It evoked considerable discussion in our course and significantly helped students to get in touch with their bodies' response to psychological or physical difficulty and healing. It also helped us activate our sensitivities to a variety of different cultural backgrounds. As the world gets smaller and more and more people come to our shores in need of sanctuary, we, as helpers, must develop greater awareness to these different responses.

Nonverbal exercises can be extremely effective during trauma and crisis for a number of reasons. By allowing the body to speak, as it were, the helplessness can be converted to empowerment. Another is that by using these techniques we can also help clients to get in touch with their bodies and to learn that there may be a pattern to the body's stress response. This learning can help the clients identify their personal "stress centers" and use them as anticipatory guidance or preventive education. Once they can recognize that part of their bodies that responds most quickly to stress, they can become aware that their stress level is starting to build up to a problematic level and take appropriate steps to reduce it. This awareness would be an indication of a new crisis situation, and by using this early warning signal clients can then apply all of the coping systems that they have learned in the present context. These exercises are another way to fill the need for the client to have something to take home from the contact with you.

In all nonverbal exercises, the helper must be aware that each individual has different areas of the body that respond to different feelings. One may experience anxiety in the neck, another in the stomach. One may harbor anger in the arms, and another may sense it in the legs. One of the author's clients was working on anger but seemed not to respond to some of the traditional anger-expressing exercises [see subsequent" Off My Back" heading]. However, whenever he seemed angered at something, his foot would kick out. Kicking exercises were designed for him, and his anger flowed easily.

The helper needs, at all times, to be observant of how the client uses the body for self-expression (Wainrib, in Wainrib & Bloch, 1998, p. 175).

Centering

This is a bioenergetic (body-mind) exercise. Stand with your feet about 10 inches apart, knees bent and toes inward, in what skiers call the snowplow position. Keeping your knees bent, allow your upper body to fall forward and over, in a downward direction, until your head is hanging down as close as possible to your feet. Breathe deeply. Using your fingertips to maintain your balance and keeping your knees bent, slowly raise your heels off the ground.

Experience the vibrations that go through your legs and into your body as you do this. Stay this way for as long as you can and then slowly return your heels to the ground, keeping your knees bent. Slowly raise your upper body to an upright position, and then raise your arms above your head. Explore the space around you with your arms and become aware of the space you own in the world. As you do this, stay in touch with your own inner center, and say, out loud if possible, "I'm alive!"

This exercise is almost as portable as the breathing. Many clients do this exercise in a variety of places, in their offices, in the cubicles of public toilets, almost anywhere. It is an excellent exercise for regaining a connection with your own center, for reducing your anxiety level, and for revitalization of energy. It gives the participant a renewed sense of power and control over one of the most essential issues in crisis intervention.

Visual Imagery

Crisis and trauma make the client feel overpowered by some enormous, uncontrollable force. Regardless of the usual coping style the client uses, increasing his or her armamentarium of skills helps to change the balance of power between the trauma and his or her own self-perception. Visual imagery, or visualization, is a simple, easy to learn skill that the practitioner can teach the client. It is another skill that the client can take along after your session.

Before you start to do imagery, it is important to have the client in a relaxed state. The progressive relaxation exercise that was described or any similar one will be helpful.

Although there are many types of visual imagery, the most important thing to remember when you are using or teaching this technique is to listen to the client's language. Some people speak very graphically and use metaphor. If so, see how you can build on their own metaphor system. For example, if a client is talking about having lost his or her footing, build your imagery around grounding, strengthening solidity, and other such concepts. If your patient is talking about feeling closed in, limited, or imprisoned, try imagery around free activity in the outdoors.

Before you start, it is often helpful to determine if the client has any phobias, dislikes, or physical limitations. For example, if your patient has a fear of skin cancer, avoid a sunny scene. If the client has a fear of height, stay away from high places.

Examples of Imagery

CLIENT (C): I'm so jittery, I can't stand it in here. I feel as if the whole world is caving in on me, and there's no place to go to.

HELPER (H): It feels like you've lost your freedom, and that is really scary.

C: Yes, and I cherish that freedom and the ability to get out and feel safe.

H: Where do you feel most free and most safe?

C: On a beach near my family's summer place.

H: Tell me about your experience of being at that place.

C: Well, it's a place where I can really unwind, and where I can really feel protected.

H: Perhaps we can go there in our minds. Close your eyes and feel yourself breathing into relaxation. Imagine your whole body gently easing up and becoming more relaxed. As you breathe comfortably, take yourself to that beach near your parents' place. Visualize yourself doing whatever you most enjoy doing at that place, perhaps walking along the shore, or watching the water, or lying on a comfortable chair or blanket.

Stay there for a while, and get a sense of how your body feels when you are there. Then think about what you are feeling and thinking. Get back in touch with who you are in that special place. See if you can take some of those feelings with you as you come back into this room.

Other examples of visual images that can be helpful in crisis or trauma include the following:

1. The swan: Allow the client to imagine herself or himself as a swan and watch the various pressures slowly roll off her or his back.
2. The skipping child: Allow the client to remember being a carefree child and reconnect to those earlier, perhaps forgotten parts.
3. The caged lion/lioness: Allow clients to visualize themselves as angry lions/lionesses in a cage may be easier for some clients than actually expressing their own anger directly.
4. Visualize oneself before this situation may help to reinstate personal empowerment. It can also function as a diagnostic tool in assessment, giving you a better image of the client's precrisis function. If this does in fact connect to a former strength, it can then be followed by visualizing oneself out of this crisis, which creates both a solution focus as well as hope.

Anger Releasing

Tailoring the anger-releasing exercise to the client's area of stress expression can be very helpful. If no such indication is given by the client, try the one that appears to be the most comfortable for both you and the client. The only caveat here is that the helper cannot be hurt by the client. Here are some examples:

Off My Back

Have the client take the same position described in the centering exercise described above. Then have the client extend the jaw, so that there is tension in the front of the neck. At the same time, have the client make two fists, raise the arms, and bend the elbows horizontally so that the fists face each other in front of the chest. Instruct the client to say, "Off my back!" loudly and vigorously as, at the same time, the client pulls his or her elbows behind him so that they try to meet behind his or her back. Do this as many times as necessary and process the exercise with the client, discussing whom he was speaking to and what unfinished business there may be that has to be addressed further.

Other Anger Exercises

Having located the client's anger center, design an exercise around that. For example, giving the client permission to stand up and stamp the floor as would a child in a tantrum can be very freeing. Having a large sturdy pillow around that the client can kick or punch is also very effective. In bioenergetics, the client is encouraged to face a couch or bed, get down on his or her knees, and strike the pillow using an entire forearm from the elbow down to the fingers. This is a far more expressive means than the usual punching and is particularly effective for women, who tend to hold their anger back at the shoulder level and are socialized to express it only in small amounts, if at all (A. Wellhaven, Personal communication, December 20, 1978).

Buckets of Paint

This is a universally used exercise that is very simple and expressively gratifying. Stand up and put your arms down alongside your body. Make a fist of both hands and imagine that in each hand you are carrying a bucket of paint. Then imagine yourself vigorously swinging the two buckets of paint back and forth and, at the same time, breathe deeply and let out a deep, guttural sound. Use your full arm, from the shoulder down, to swing the buckets.

Positive Reinforcers

People in crisis need now more than at any other time to take care of themselves, but, by the very nature of the experience, they may generally do very little self-care. It is therefore important for you to set up "goody contracts" with the client. These involve first letting clients tell you some of the things that they can do to feel good. These might include taking a long quiet tub bath, eating a candy bar, going for a quiet walk, having a good meal, watching the clouds drift across the quiet sky, having a quiet cup of herbal tea, or any number of things that clients may suggest. Each of these suggestions may sound like an anathema to you if you are picturing people staying at a shelter in the midst of a natural disaster, but that is exactly what makes the reinforcers so precious and important. Then set up a contract with them in which they agree to do (or try to do) at least one of these take-care-of-yourself things before your next meeting. If clients have a particularly difficult task to do, you can do a variation of the goody contract by helping them to chunk the task into small, "doable" pieces, and then, after each piece, to reward themselves with one of the things on their goody contract list.

Sleep Exercises

A recent review of psychological treatments for insomnia (Murtagh & Greenwood, 1995) has shown that these techniques are effective treatments for improving sleep patterns and subjective experience of sleep. Because crisis and trauma produce sleep deprivation, we report some of this work here. The treatments examined in the study were stimulus control, sleep restriction, paradoxical intent, and relaxation techniques. Stimulus control techniques focus on being in bed only when one is sleepy. "Clients are instructed to use the bedroom only for sleep and sex and not for reading, watching television, eating, or working." They are further instructed to "get out of bed when they are unable to sleep and to get out of bed at the same time every morning regardless of the amount of sleep" (Murtagh & Greenwood, 1995, p. 82).

Other relaxation techniques useful for promoting sleep include progressive muscle relaxation, meditation, systematic desensitization, imagery, autogenic training, and hypnosis. Our own work has found that the cognitive therapy concept of "thought stoppage" can be very helpful, particularly for constricted clients who ruminate about a troubling situation and have difficulty in moving on. For those who have sleep difficulties related to a trauma, a simple method that I have found effective for quieting the mind is to have the client find a seven-syllable set of letters or numbers, or a phrase that she or he can repeat over and over again. The Canadian postal-code system provides an excellent choice for this, and it can be shared with anyone. The postal code seems to have the correct number of syllables and has been used effectively by many. An example of this is H3W2Y4. Another peace-inspiring, mantra-like phrase that has been found to be helpful is "the grass grows all by itself," or, for winter lovers, "the snow falls all by itself."

REFERENCES

Louden, J. (1992). *The woman's comfort book* (pp. 18, 49). San Francisco: Harper.

Lowen A. (1976). *Depression and the body*. England: Penguin Books.

Lowen, A., & Lowen, L. (1977). *The way to vibrant health: A manual of bioenergetic exercise*. New York: Harper Colophon.

Murtagh, D. R., & Greenwood K .M. (1995). Identifying effective psychological treatments for insomnia: A meta-analysis. *Journal of Consulting and Clinical Psychology, 63,* 79–89.

Rosenbloom, D., & Williams, M. (1999). *Life after trauma: A workbook for healing.* New York: Guilford Press

Rothschild, B. (2000). *The body remembers* (pp. 5–6, 100). New York: W.W. Norton & Co.

Van der Kolk, B. (2004, January). *Psychotherapy Networker,* 35.

Wainrib, B., in B. Wainrib & E. Bloch. (1998). *Crisis intervention and trauma response: Theory and practice.* New York: Springer Publishing.

CHAPTER 9

Spirituality and Trauma

Soul holds together mind and body, ideas and life, spirituality and the world.
                            —Marsilio Ficino (15th century)

Everyone who is seriously involved in the pursuit of science becomes convinced that a Spirit is manifest in the Laws of the Universe.
                            —Albert Einstein (20th century)

DEFINING AND UNDERSTANDING SPIRITUALITY'S ROLE IN TRAUMA

In "Spirituality and Trauma: An Essay," Robert Grant, PhD (1999), writes: "Traumatic experiences force victims to face issues lying outside the boundaries of personal and collective frames of reference. As a result, they are forced to confront psychological and spiritual challenges that are unfamiliar to the average person. . . . Trauma is life at its worst." All of us who have worked in this area will recognize that description. Grant adds:

> Traumatic events are often unexpected and horrible. Typically they lead to a variety of physical, emotional interpersonal and spiritual problems. . . . Most victims feel lost, disoriented and powerless when former ways of making their bearings have been damaged or destroyed. . . . Many lose their bearings. . . . Many wander indefinitely until new and more comprehensive ways of taking up life are created. . . . Old ways of understanding are exposed as inadequate. Trying to ignore the profound shifts occurring in consciousness is not without cost.

121

Grant introduces a more positive note: "Trauma, in spite of its brutality and destructiveness, has the power to open victims to issues of profound existential and spiritual significance. (Trauma) throws victims onto a path that mystics, shamans, mythic heroes and spiritual seekers have been walking for thousands of years."

Grant concludes, "If health is to be restored then the help of the Spirit and others is required. Acknowledging this *fundamental dependency* is a critical milestone on the healing path" (p. 25).

Dr. Grant's words were borne out in reality following the horrors of September 11, 2001 (9-11), which produced an immediate increase in people's interest both in personal spirituality and in organized religion. A story in a Toronto newspaper, the *Globe and Mail* (September 13, 2001), told of a man who miraculously escaped from the World Trade Tower. The reporter says, "Even though he was unharmed, Mr. F. says he was changed by the experience. Normally not a particularly religious man, he recalls that as he prepared for bed at his home on the night of September 11, he looked out his window and saw a huge buck deer on his lawn. The deer turned and stared at him. 'It was like I was looking into God's eyes,' he said: 'And He was looking into my soul. He (God) was saying to me 'if you thought you were alone, you weren't. I was with you every step of the way.'" He reports that he found himself increasingly involved in his religious practices and continued them as of the time of the interview.

Mr. F. is not alone in his reaction. Fourteen million visitors were registered for online prayer groups in Canada in the month after 9-11. Patrick Brethour, technology reporter of the *Globe and Mail* (National newspaper in Canada) reported on Wednesday, November 14, 2001, that "patriotism and prayer have sent Web traffic in the United States soaring to record levels as Americans search for outlets to express their solidarity in the face of terrorism and war" (p. 16). Jupiter Media Matrix Inc. said that its "traffic figures for October show a clear shift since September in the surfing inclinations of Americans away from news and charity sites and toward those that give them an outlet for patriotism or spirituality. . . . Americans . . . turned to spiritual sources of inspiration" (2001).

Our vision of the world and the impact it has had on our sense of security has changed dramatically since 9-11. Each of us, in our own way, have an increased sense of personal vulnerability, and many of us, in the privacy of our homes, may be repeating Mr. F's reaction and seeking spiritual connectedness.

Drescher and Foy, in an article titled "Spirituality and Trauma Treatment" (1995), tell us: "There is an increasing recognition that many patients view spirituality as a primary human dimension. Indeed current concepts of coping strategies are evolving to include spiritual beliefs and practices along with other social, physical and cognitive aspects, as important coping resources."

They continue, "Traumatic events often lead to dramatic changes in survivors' world views so that fundamental assumptions about meaningfulness, goodness, and safety shift negatively. For those whose core values are theologically founded, traumatic events often give rise to questions about the fundamental nature of the relationship between the creator and humankind."

Drescher and Foy report that "in a recent study it was suggested that religiously committed women who are battered suffer less severe PTSD symptoms than women without such commitment" (p. 236). Linley (2004), in an article called "Positive Change Following Trauma and Adversity," found that "religious activities and intrinsic religiousness were both positively related with growth after trauma" (p. 16).

Janice Goldfein, a psychotherapist, reports that she used religious rituals in helping to heal from her rape experience:

> I knew there were several religious rituals that could promote healing and
> help me move beyond the horror and revulsion of the sexual assault. . . .
> Whenever Jews survive a life-threatening event, they are obligated to re-
> cite a prayer of gratitude. . . . Following the attack, I stood on the women's
> side of the of the synagogue and recited "Blessed art thou our God, King
> of the universe, who bestows favors and hast shown me kindness (2004).

The entire congregation then responded to her with a similar statement.

She reports, "I felt a tremendous sense of support from my community and a profound gratitude for my survival." She also reports that she had been gagging and unable to swallow from the time of the rape, but subsequently went through a ritual bath and reports that "It freed me from that sense of defilement and returned me to a sense of my own holiness" (Personal communication, 2003).

In a study of practitioners conducted by the Practice Directorate of the American Psychological Association (APA) shortly after 9-11, 48% of the respondents reported that they had used spiritual and/or religious involvement as a strategy for dealing with their own reactions to the 9-11 disaster.

Barrett (1999) tells us that "the healing from trauma is a quest for spirituality." Barrett has developed a model of recovery that happens in stages. "First is acknowledgment, in a safe environment, how the trauma has impacted the spirit; acknowledging how you have changed and rekindling the desire to spiritually reconnect with self and other. Next, design of the personal training program that will recreate the proactive energy which lies within all of us."

Barrett (1999) further explains, "During this stage comes the spiritual practice that will take out personal vibrations and continue to build energy. Finally, we take the commitment to ongoing spiritual practice-commitment to continue doing something different, building on compassion morality and kindness toward self and community" (p. 95).

THERAPEUTIC SPIRITUALITY: APPLYING SPIRITUALITY TO TRAUMATIC SITUATIONS

The concept of spirituality and spiritual practice, particularly as it relates to psychotherapeutic practice, can raise eyebrows amongst many people, whether clients, colleagues or helpers. However, spiritual connections may often emerge spontaneously in our work with traumatized people. Although I never plan it, I often find that when I am truly working in synchronicity with clients, both the client and myself will experience a deeply spiritual connection which is always extremely moving for both of us and frequently leads to important growth for the client.

One example of this follows: I had been working with a very special woman for some time. A successful mental health practitioner, she had suffered from extremely severe childhood trauma, which had been deeply suppressed for much of her life. After attaining considerable success in her chosen field, she started to have flashbacks of delayed memories of the horrors, which had never before been revealed until she came to work with me. Many of our sessions achieved the sense of deep connectedness referred to previously.

As we reached the end of one session, suddenly she suggested that she needed to join in some kind of organized prayer expression. Prayer is not anything that I traditionally do in my practice, yet I felt comfortable with her suggestion. Since we both come from very different religious backgrounds, we tried to find a common prayer. Finally, I asked her if she was familiar with what, in Hebrew, is the *Priest's Prayer*, which exists in the Christian liturgy as well:

> "May the Lord bless thee and keep thee
> May the Lord cause his countenance to shine upon thee (etc.)"

She agreed and asked if we could say it together. We said it together in English, our common language, and as we did, I felt a sense of something much greater enter the room, but I did not mention it. After we finished, she asked me what I had experienced during the prayer. When I asked her what prompted her question, she responded that it was because she could see something come over me that changed my appearance. Then I told her that something I could not name seemed to enter the room and come over me. We both sat in silence for a while, but it was a very special, intense, open, connected silence—the kind that we have in many therapy sessions when we have come into soul-to-soul contact.

This woman had visited me from another country, and after she got home, she wrote to me and said that even though she had never previously given me this information, the particular prayer that I had chosen was the one that she had used to survive throughout her very painful childhood. Saying the prayer together was an intensely spiritual and meaningful experience for her, as well as for me. The experience gave her a renewed sense of healing. If you ask me for directions in evoking this sense, I will have to confess that I cannot give them to you. This woman and I had worked together for a long time and had built up an important connection with each other, one that both permitted as well as helped to create this deeply healing and, spiritual experience.

How do we create the essence of spirituality in therapy with traumatized people? What must we explore and experience within ourselves and our clients to reach this goal?

In order to approach some of these questions we must first add some additional ones. Many of us would agree that the concept of spirituality is closely related with the concept of "soul." As Thomas Moore (the contemporary one) said in *Care of the Soul* (1992): "Soul is not a thing but a quality or dimension of experiencing life and ourselves. It has to do with depth, value, relatedness, heart and personal substance" (p. 9). Psychologist David Elkins, past president of the Division of Humanistic Psychology of the APA, has written a fascinating book called *Beyond Religion* (1998). My meeting him was one of those chance meetings of kindred souls. I was in California where, at the California School of Professional Psychology, I was teaching a postgraduate course titled "Crisis and Trauma," and he was one of my students. At the end of the course, he struck up an interesting conversation with me and gave me a copy of his book. I have found the book of great value in my own search of this topic, and I would recommend it highly. In his chapter titled "The Soul-Doorway to the Imaginal World," he tells us the following:

> According to an old Hindu legend there was once a time when all human beings were Gods but they so abused their divinity that Brahma, the chief God decided to take it away from them and hide it where it could never

be found. Where to hide their divinity was the question. So Brahma called a council of the gods to help him decide. "Lets bury it deep in the earth," said the gods. But Brahma answered, "No, that will not do because humans will dig deep within the earth and find it." The gods said, "Lets sink it deep in the ocean." And Brahma answered "No, not there for they will learn to dive into the ocean and will find it." The gods said "Let's take it to the top of the highest mountain." And Brahma said, "No, not there because they will eventually climb every mountain and once again take up their divinity." Then the gods gave up and said "We do not know where to hide it because it seems that there is no place on earth or in the sea that human beings will not eventually reach." Brahma thought for a long time and then said "Here is what we will do: We will hide their divinity deep in the center of their own being, for humans will never think to look for it there." All the gods agreed that that was the perfect hiding place and the deed was done. And since then, human beings have been going up and down the earth digging, diving, climbing, and exploring, searching for something that is already within themselves (p. 37).

Elkins (1998) also tells us that the word psychology comes from two Greek words—psyche and logos. Psyche means "soul" and logo, in this context, means "study." Thus, the word psychology essentially means "the study of the soul." In the same way, Elkins tells us, other key words in the field, also point to the soul. For example, the word "therapist" meant "servant" or "attendant." Thus, entomologically, a psychotherapist is a servant or attendant of the soul. The word psychopathology has a similar root. The Greek words psyche and pathos literally mean the "suffering of the soul." Hence, each of us in the helping professions, particularly in psychotherapy, are automatically the keepers of the souls of those who seek our help. Therefore, delving into the soul of psychotherapy is not just a luxury or an intellectual exercise. It is a part of our basic training in the helping professions.

Whether or not we respect that obligation will depend upon many things, as we shall soon see. For many of us, the concept of true connection is perhaps easier to accept than its definition as soul. True connection is not an act of intellectual distance or theory, nor is it a distant pretense; it reflects our individual abilities to open our own hearts and souls to another. Although, more often than not, human connection with other humans uses that model as a constant in our lives, often in times of crisis or trauma, what is visible to us is *not* connections, but dissonance, pain, and hurt. Trauma in itself not only severs connections but it damages our ability to trust others and allow ourselves to become vulnerable. This vulnerability can, in return, act as a beacon of spiritual connection.

How do we start to create this connection, this sense of the soul within and between ourselves? Years ago when I was running groups for college students, I asked them to write something in any medium that expressed their experience.

One of the poems that was given to me said, quite simply, "In the warmth of this circle when our souls touch I know who I can be."

These lines stay with me, for in their simplicity they tell us much about the question we have just posed.

If we do start to understand the concept of spirituality and spiritual connection, how do we create the sense of the intense connectedness that it seems to imply? What is the connection between soul and spirituality? How can we allow ourselves the enormous risk of souls touching if one or both of us have been traumatized? And how do we define spirituality in general? Elkins (1998) tells us "Carl Jung was the first psychologist to recognize the importance of the soul and make it a major psychological construct. While Freud had little interest in spirituality and even considered it a sign of neurosis, Jung made spirituality the center of his therapeutic work and believed the recovery of the soul was essential for both the individual and western society" (p. 20).

Jung's work is now experiencing a revival, and Jungian themes such as "archetypes, mythology, spirituality, and the soul are being discussed widely . . . and attracting the attention of millions" (Elkins, p. 20).

We all have our own definition of concepts like soul and spirituality, which is fine as long as we agree to disagree occasionally. In trying to connect these two words, soul and spirit, and to connect these mysteries, we can call again on Elkins (1998), who tells us that "spirituality, which comes from the Latin "spiritus" meaning "breath of life," is a way of being and experiencing that comes about through awareness of a transcendent dimension and that is characterized by certain identifiable values in regard to self, others, nature life and whatever one considers to be the Ultimate" (p. 26).

There are numerous approaches and definitions to this intellectually very complicated, yet emotionally understandable, concept. When you approach an ordinary dictionary for a definition of the word "spirituality," you get a bit of a runaround. Webster's says, "pertaining to or consisting of spirit or incorporeal being; or pertaining to the spirit or to the soul as distinguished from the physical nature; or pertaining to the spirit as in the seat of moral or religious nature, symbolic or mystical -also religious, devotional or sacred [etc]."

There is a vagueness, an ambiguity about this concept. For example, the Dalai Lama (1991) says the following:

> What I call basic spirituality are the basic human qualities of goodness, kindness, compassion, and caring. Whether we are believers or non-believers this kind of spirituality is essential. As long as we are human beings, as long as we are members of the human family all of us need these basic spiritual values. We must still find a way to try to improve life for the majority of the people.

Think briefly about how you, the reader, would define this important but amorphous concept. Elkins (1998) tells us that "spirituality is the process and result of nurturing the soul and developing one's spiritual life. While many do this in the context of traditional religion it must be recognized that religion is only one path to spiritual development and that there are may be alternative paths as well" (p. 20).

As therapists, we are healers. We do not practice with medical instruments or medications. Unfortunately, however, there are times when we become overinvolved in our work or fail to recognize our own exhaustion. These are behaviors that threaten the maintenance of our own strengths. For some of us, this may appear to be developing greater understanding in our work. For others, however, it creates the threat of diminishing their gift of healing. At these times, we are vulnerable to becoming "wounded healers." Dr. Joy Dunkin (2002), as well as others, reminds us that "Carl Jung's archetype of the 'Wounded Healer' originated with the Greek myth of Chiron, who was physically wounded, and by way of overcoming the pain of his own wounds, Chiron became the compassionate teacher of healing." We must learn, however, that overcoming our pain is not achieved by taking on more than we can carry.

Our greatest gift to each other is the essence of sharing our souls and validating what emerges from our clients' souls. Thus, we need not only to stay in touch with our souls, but to understand them as well. In order to do that, we may find it helpful to define our own personal meaning for spirituality.

Each of us has his or her own personal language of spirituality. To identify that language, first an individual must understand what nourishes his or her own spirit and/or soul, and then, he or she must respect the variety of means in which he or she can touch that soul.

The following is my definition of spirituality: A quality of true connectedness, which we shall refer to as "communion," a coming together with an "other," is for me the essence of spirituality. This element of coming in close contact with an "other," whether it be a thing, a person, an animal, or an idea, is part of every spiritual experience. And that same communion, that coming together, is the essence of healing. Although we are born alone and die alone, much of our lifetime quest is to reconnect with some lost attachment. Whether this attachment is the Garden of Eden or one's mother's womb, that sense of loss is part of the human condition. Wholeness—a sense of being healed—is the satisfaction of that quest, an experience of being reconnected. Trauma takes that sense of connectedness away from us. It makes us feel isolated from the rest of the world, alone, and terrified.

Nevertheless, we can experience communion in a wide variety of ways, from the mundane to the sublime. For example, when we allow ourselves to laugh with someone else, we are acknowledging that we are on the same wave length, that we see the world together, that we are "in synch." We are no longer alone. We feel whole. It is no surprise, then, that laughter has been shown to be a healing experience in life-threatening illness.

When trauma or any kind of crisis strikes, not only are we separated from some "other," but we feel different from everyone else in our world. We can create a "oneness" with another person or group, or with a memory of an experience, or with an emotion, or with a higher power.

If we are fortunate enough to experience the "oneness" with another person, we have engaged in what Martin Buber (1958) called an "I-Thou" relationship. Going beyond ourselves and our loneliness can help us to feel whole. The Zen philosophy is based on the concept of giving up our preoccupation with ourselves and becoming one with whatever we are doing, whether this be skiing, praying, or doing motorcycle maintenance. This, too, takes us beyond our loneliness.

When our "oneness" is with a higher power, that power may be experienced as either outside of or within ourselves. Either way, it gives us a sense of being completely understood, completely connected, in communion with something.

In the traditional Judeo-Christian religions, the God image is one that not only make us whole but also evokes a protectedness that brings back memories of the Eden/Womb. When we experience this sense of connection and communion, we are experiencing our spirituality. This quality of connectedness can also come from a moment with nature. The perfect stillness of the woods in winter, the awe of the moment as a single drop of snow falls from a tree limb, the constant flow of a brook, the unique beauty of a flower—all of these carry with them a sense of breathlessness that takes us in and includes us in something larger than ourselves. At a purely logical level, we recognize our minuteness in the face of nature's vastness. Yet, in these moments of awe, we sense a communion that includes us in nature's beauty, and we are no longer alone.

All of these experiences—laughter, being "in synch," interpersonal intimacy, connection with an internal or external "higher power," a moment in nature—are healing experiences. All serve to eradicate our isolation and help us to feel reconnected with that lost "other." This reconnection, this communion, is a spiritual healing. In order to have these experiences, we have to be open to them. We have to allow ourselves to realize that we are, in reality, in search of some completion. Yes, we are competent, well functioning adults who are independent in many ways. Acknowledging this incomplete part of ourselves opens us to the enriching of our being, to feel fully alive and to be healed. When we talk of "getting in touch with our spirituality" or "exploring our spirituality," we are acknowledging our openness to explore that need for completion.

As individual and diverse as our various and varied definitions of spirituality may be, we must also heed the words of Joseph Campbell (1973):

> There is a thought that I have long and faithfully entertained: of the unity of the race of man, not only in its biology, but also in its spiritual history, which has everywhere unfolded in the manner of a single symphony, with its themes announced developed, amplified and turned about, distorted, reasserted, and today in a grand fortissimo of all sections standing together irresistibly advancing to some kind of a mighty climax out of which the next great movement will emerge (p. 205).

And, applying these concepts to our own work, let us remember David Elkins (1998) once more, who tells us that "Counseling and psychotherapy are ways to nurture the soul, roads to a deeper spiritual life: I take seriously the idea that psychopathology is the suffering of the soul and that therapy is the cure and care of the soul" (p. 175). We must also understand that our spiritual selves, as our beings themselves, are not always radiant and joyous. Sometimes we hear of the struggle of the "dark night of the soul." Perhaps we need some understanding of the darkness and the light in our lives and how that hurts or enriches our souls.

All of us in the helping professions know that as much as we can relish the times of connectedness and brightness, many of us will often and sometimes frequently experience periods of darkness. We also know, unfortunately, that some people experience lives of darkness.

It is not just external circumstances that bring us darkness. Our own bodies can and do provide similar threats, as we have already seen in chapter 5. We can also each create our own darkness in our failures at connection with each other, even in the best-intentioned relationship. However, when we have also experienced times of joy and contact, we learn that, we can move through those times of darkness. We sometimes even learn that, with the right ingredients, such as social support and understanding, we can use that darkness as a stage toward growth and choice.

If we understand the paradigm of change developed long ago by Van Gennep (1960), then we can learn that its stages include mourning, confusion, and reemergence. At a time when we have suffered any kind of life transition, crisis, or trauma, our psyches need first to mourn for the fact that, whether for better or for worse, our lives will never be the same. Then, we need to allow ourselves to experience and recognize the confusion of knowing who we were but not knowing who we will be; eventually, there will be a reemergence of our selves and our souls in a new sense of identity. As it is very difficult to feel "open" during the periods of the dark night of the soul, it is particularly important for the helping professional to be sensitive to the process that this darkness opens. Darkness is often the path of life transitions. It represents a necessary loss in our lives.

As we go through life, many of us will encounter crisis or trauma. Some of the crises may have a very different connotation from trauma; they may be crises of growth, such as marriage, or the birth of a child. In spite of their surface joy, they represent a loss, a loss of how things were before the transition occurred. Even though the change may bring joy, it also heralds a time when life will never again be the same as it had been. And strange as it may seem, we have the right to mourn the loss of life as it was because it is now changed and gone.

In the darkness of trauma, all of the human being, body, mind, and soul have been robbed of comfort, security, predictability. All of our stabilities have been shaken or lost. What we have left is primarily our inner spirit, our essential beliefs. Hence, the next aspect of the spirit's dark night is a searching—a searching through a time of confusion, of knowing how we were but without a clear road map or path to where we may be going. We are searching at these times for a new definition of ourselves. Our lives have changed and our spirits, somehow, may be aware of that much sooner than our brains. Finally, the dark night starts to brighten again, the dawn gradually develops, and from it comes a clearer sense of who we are, a new self, a new identity, a new form of spirituality leading to a soul that is at peace with the new self.

If we help the client by focusing on the potential for growth rather than on the sense of despair, we can become midwives to the emergence of newness. We must remember, however, that it is there, in the darkness and the turmoil, in the confusion—it is there that the process of change emerges— and it is in those places where our interventions can be of most value. This is the process that we need to shepherd as we watch the individual's soul go through the struggles of changes that come either internally or externally to our lives.

Many of us have seen people who appear to be living neither in the true depths of the darkness nor in the brightness of the light, people for whom the spark of soul appears to be missing. They go through the routine motions of their day but do not savor what life really has to offer. Their days come and go, and they often fail to experience the warmth of the sunshine or the smell of fresh cut grass, or the colors of the autumn leaves. In the over 40 years that I have been privileged to work in my professional field, I have seen that the ability to choose a soul-satisfying life is almost as fragile as life itself. At any point along our life cycle, from conception on, genetics, abuse, chemical imbalances, emotional pain, depression, trauma, loss, misunderstandings, and many other sources of distress can deprive our souls of the full richness of life. Some people's pain is so great that they struggle daily with the decision to choose life. Unfortunately, I also know those who wish they could choose life but whose time is shortened by degenerative disease or life-threatening illness. So we cannot take a full soul-centered life for granted.

The great Christian theologian Paul Tillich (1966), in his writings in *The Shaking of Foundations,* describes some of the process of this pain and its need for soul healing. He says,

> Grace strikes us when we are in great pain and restlessness. It strikes us when we walk through the dark valley of a meaningless and empty life. It strikes us when we feel that our separation is deeper than usual, because we have violated another life, a life which we loved or from whom we were estranged (p. 184).

It strikes us when our disgust for our own being, our indifference, our weakness, our hostility, and our lack of direction and composure have become intolerable to us. It strikes us when, year after year, the longed-for perfection of life does not appear; when the old compulsions reign within us as they have for decades, when despair destroys all joy and courage. Sometimes at that moment, a wave of life breaks into the darkness, and it is as though a voice were saying, "You are accepted. You are accepted, accepted by that which is greater than you and the name of which you do not know" (Elkins, 1998, p. 184).

Much of our role is in helping those people recognize the message of "you are accepted" by ourselves, by the world, by whatever spiritual belief they may have—and, ultimately the most difficult, acceptance by themselves as the person they have become, reemerging from their traumatic experience.

But often more than not, what we see in our professional lives is the pain of those of our clients, who often have difficulty in truly choosing life, who have not been able to allow themselves to truly heal, who do not believe that they are entitled to acceptance. But here, too, our own experience of soul comes forth. Because it is when we are fully in touch with our own souls that we can truly connect with the souls of those who are in pain and who are experiencing a sense of being lost, a sense of being out of touch with their souls.

So it is incumbent upon us in the healing professions to connect with and maintain connection with our own souls.

And what do we need to know in order to stay in touch with our souls? Quoting Elkins (1998) again:

> The raw material of soul making is ontos—"being": and in doing therapy I have often had the sense that I am working with ontological clay, that the client's being is emerging and that the client and I, like two sculptors are gently molding, shaping and working it until it takes form. . . . Just as the creative artist must follow his intuitive sense to produce the work of art, the creative therapist must follow the authentic nature and emergence of the client's being in order to help it become what it is trying to become (p. 182).

Although the soul and the spirit are not bound to any religious group, each religion has made has made contributions to our understanding of them. Recent research by Dr. Elizabeth Targ has shown that people who have a spiritual practice or who subscribe to religious denominations tend to experience less distress in the face of calamity, to live longer, and to recover faster from illness (2002). As practitioners, we need to be aware of this, if we have not yet been, and we must be prepared to deal with the soul connection that this kind of disruption can create. Others have emphasized that human connectedness in the key.

Levine and Levine (1995) tell us that (interpersonal) "relationships offer pathways for spiritual growth as they strengthen resilience, as in the Quaker adage "I lift thee and thou lifts me."

Caring bonds with partners, family members, and close friends nourish spiritual well being; in turn, spirituality deepens and expands our connections with others. It can be a spiritual experience to share physical and emotional angers or to receive the loving kindness of other.

How can we as mere mortal therapists initiate the creation of that voice of acceptance, of grace, that connection or reconnection with the soul of someone who is a "lost soul"? We certainly cannot do that if we do not nourish our own souls.

Again, David Elkins (1998) tells us how the therapist can create this kind of moment: He says, "Therapist congruence—the alignment of the therapist's outward behavior with her inner experience—is ontological in nature in that the therapist is in contact with her own being and is thereby bringing authentic being to the therapeutic encounter." Elkins (1998) continues, "In the presence of an authentic therapist the client's being no matter how repressed will resonate and respond" (p. 168).

Of course, essential to all this work is the ability to be a truly caring, professional listener. Remember that the Chinese symbol for listening is "ears, eyes, heart." Perhaps when we do that we will experience "the warmth of this circle—where our souls touch, and we know who we are."

REFERENCES

Barrett, M. J. (1999). Walsh, F. (Ed.) *Spiritual resources in family therapy* (p. 95). New York: Guilford.

Brethour, P. (2001, November 14). The *Globe and Mail* (Toronto, Canada).

Buber, M. (1958). *I and thou*. New York: Scribner.

Campbell, J. (1973). *Myths to live by*. New York: Bantam Books.

Dalai Lama. (1991). The Tibet Center, New York.

Drescher, K. D., & Foy, D. W. (1995). Spirituality and trauma treatment: Suggestions for including spirituality as a coping resource. *NCP Clinical Quarterly, 5*(1).

Dunkin, J. (2002). "The Wounded Healer." Retrieved from http://www.awakening-healing.com/AHNewsLetters/2002/Mercury&Chrion.htm.

Einstein, A. (1979). Dukas, H. & Hoffman, B. (Eds.), *Albert Einstein, The human side*. Princeton, NJ: Princeton University Press.

Elkins, D. (1998). *Beyond religion*. Wheaton, IL: Theosophical Publishing House.

Ficino, M. (1975). *The letters of Marsilio Ficino* (vol. 1). London: Fellowship of the School of Economic Science.

Goldfein, J. (2004). Reclaiming the self. *Psychotherapy Networker, 2,* 47, 52.

Grant, R. (1999). Spirituality and trauma: An essay. *Traumatology, 5*(1E2) (abstract).

Jupiter Media Matrix Inc. November 20, 2001. Radio information.

Levine, S., & Levine, O. (1995). *Relationship as a path of awakening*. Dublin, Ireland: Gill & Macmillan Ltd.

Linley, J. (2004). Positive change following trauma and adversity. *Journal of Traumatic Stress, 17*(1), 16.

Moore, T. (1992). *Care of the soul*. New York: Harper Collins Publishers.

Targ, E. (2002, Spring). Seven reasons we may live longer. *Spirituality and Health*.

Tillich, P., cited in Elkins, D. (1998). *Beyond religion*. Wheaton, IL: Theosophical Publishing House.

Van Gennep, A. (1960). *Rites of passage*. Chicago: University of Chicago Press.

Wainrib, B. (2002, May 16). "Counseling Soul to Soul." Keynote address. Canadian Counseling Association, Annual Meeting, Ottawa, Canada.

CHAPTER 10

New Sources of Healing

Love cures people, both the ones who give it and the ones who receive it.
—Dr. Karl Menninger (1893–1990)

HEALING THE HEALERS:
ASSESSING YOUR OWN RESOURCES

As you have read through this book, you may have been doing a personal assessment of your own resources in each situation that has been presented. You may have found yourself wondering if you have the resources necessary to truly respond appropriately for yourself or to aid a client. Some aspects of our resource bank have not yet been touched upon, and this chapter's goal is to expand your thinking about some of the as yet unmentioned resources, particularly as they apply to the new world in which we now find ourselves.

DEFINING HEALING

What do you think of when you hear the word "healing"? Does it relate only to your body, or to your very being? Can you remember times in your life when your body was totally intact, and yet you felt ripped apart internally?

Healing involves actively pursuing a personal sense of "wholeness" so that you come to feel more and more connected to your innermost self and to the life you are leading. It does not mean putting your life on hold, waiting for something to happen that will force the connection. To sustain the process of healing you must listen to what your heart and soul have to say which may require studying their language with new intensity (Wainrib & Haber, 2000, p. 248).

Healing refers to external relationships as well as internally, to our bodies and our souls. Do not forget the healing power of relationships. In particular, remember that, in the final analysis, resiliency flourishes in acts of caring for each other.

REACHING OUT TO COMMUNITIES: USING THE MEDIA IN HEALING POLITICAL UNREST—THE QUEBEC REFERENDUM AND THE ANGLOPHONE COMMUNITY

For many of our readers, Canada is that very cold country to the north. It is generally seen as a peaceful country that has much less political upheaval than does the United States. This location was chosen to demonstrate the use of the media primarily because it is truly a peaceful country most of the time. It is presented here to describe a situation of potential mass trauma that was dealt with in an unusual manner.

While North Americans may experience much excitement around political elections, neither trauma, political turmoil, nor community crisis are words we generally associate with these experiences. In 1995, in Quebec, some of its ethnic groups experienced not only political unrest but reactions that elicited reawakening of earlier traumatic experiences, both personal and collective. This chapter will describe the experience and ways in which psychologists were able to make use of the media to respond to this mass reaction.

Brief Historical Background

Canada was founded by two distinct ethnic groups, the English and the French. Because of an unfortunate experience on the Plains of Abraham in the 18th century, a true integration of these two groups has been hard to establish. I will spare you the details, but, suffice it to say that, until the late 1960s, the majority of the Province of Quebec was French (by birth, culture, and language) while the province's political power was in the hands of the English.

The election of 1968 changed all of that. The Lesage government came into office with the slogan *maîtres chez nous,* masters in our own house. Enormous reforms in the educational system (which had been under religious control), as well as the health care system, brought the province into greater synchrony with the rest of North America. The Church's hold on education and the people was weakened, and postsecondary education emphasized more pragmatic subjects. Years of political suppression awakened a smoldering sense of national pride in the hearts of the predominantly French population, awakening a long suppressed, passionate need for an identity that was separate from that of the rest of Canada. The threat that it posed to the traditional original English-speaking population created a mass exodus from the province. A third force, people who were emigrating from beleaguered parts of the world seeking a sense of safety, and often having experienced considerable trauma, largely replaced those who had moved away. The population that left were, by and large, replaced by this third force in the scenario, labeled "Allophones." Gradually, different voices, different clothing, and different cultures became more visible in the province.

By 1976, the spirit of nationalism and individual identity was strong enough to elect the first government of the *Parti Québecois,* the Quebec Party, whose goal, as chanted the night of the election was *Québec pour les Québecois,* Quebec for true, that is, original, Quebecers. Its underlying goal was to separate from the rest of Canada. This government brought with them further reforms in the educational system and a strong emphasis on the need for use of, and respect for, the French language. French became the official language of work and the *Office de la Langue Francais,* the "language police," was created to supervise this. Routine visits from this authority affirmed that French was being used as the language of work. All of this made a certain sense since the French were the majority of the population and had been ignored for far too long.

In a fairly short time, many of the original goals appeared to have been reached: businesses and professions were now run primarily by Francophones. The province was now, in reality to most outsiders, what its founders had originally dreamt of.

As each of these reforms took place, there was an exodus of Anglophones and Allophones (comfortably bilingual people) who were concerned about their future security. This in itself is an aberration. Canada, unlike the United States, is not a transient society. People live in the same places as did their parents and grandparents, and, generally speaking, students who do leave to go away to school, do it at the graduate and not the undergraduate level. Support systems are generally family-oriented, and each exodus began a breakdown of naturally occurring psychological support.

In 1984, the proseparatist government then in power felt it was time to hold a second referendum to secede from Canada. The issue was no longer just language. Negotiations with the other provinces had failed to assure Quebec of recognition as a distinct society. As the days came closer to the referendum, it seemed as if separation might really happen. A rally of 100,000 people from all over Canada was held 2 days before the election to support the "non" campaign—the campaign that believed in federalism and was saying no" to separatism.

The Referendum

On October 31, 1995, the referendum was held. The results came in slowly, with the earlier results coming from outside of Montreal. The final result was 49.5 % for separation, 50.5 % for remaining in a federal Canada.

The results, followed by some unfortunate statements in the losing party, contributed even further to the reactivation of the many who had migrated to Canada in search of political safety, as well as that part of the population that had experienced politically oriented trauma in their former countries of residences who had calmly assumed that no such thing could ever happen in their homeland. Living in an unstable political environment with a visible threat of being victimized can establish a potential sensitivity for trauma as well as easily reactivate former experiences of politically created trauma.

For weeks before the actual vote, almost every one of my therapy patients (all English-speaking, many comfortably bilingual) would make some reference to their growing anxiety about the election. They reported serious concerns about their personal welfare, their future in a separate Quebec, fears about their money being frozen or devalued, fears for loss of their property value, loss of family and friends who would move, and other such issues. A psychoanalytic colleague of mine described similar experience in her practice. She said, "There is no interpretation—it's all reality anxiety." People who I met in the community were reporting the same fears.

Whether or not this scene would be experienced by an outsider as true political unrest, what had started out as a completely democratic election was now being experienced by a large part of the population as the beginnings of political unrest, and they were, in turn, reacting with symptoms that one would rarely expect to see in this population. Many of the newer groups of immigrants had come to Canada to escape past experiences of psychological and physical abuse in their home countries. *MacLean's Magazine,* a national magazine in Canada, referred to the situation as "Anglo Angst."

On the night after the election, I met with the 40 plus students in my graduate course, called "Crisis and Trauma," at McGill University. These students came from every one of the groups we described. Although many were from old Canadian families, both Anglophone and Francophone, a large group represented the new immigrants, the Allophones. I was then in the midst of writing a book, *Crisis Intervention and Trauma Response: Theory and Practice* (Wainrib & Bloch, 1998), and I was using part of it for the course. After a general discussion of the students' reactions to the situation, I suggested that they look back at chapter 3 and an adaptation of Framer's (1990) list of "most common symptoms" of posttraumatic stress. These symptoms were

- emotional numbing
- disbelief
- sleep disturbances, nightmares, night terrors in children
- anger and irritability
- flashbacks, intrusive thoughts
- sadness
- forgetfulness and loss of concentration
- fears of "going crazy"
- survivor guilt
- loss of feeling secure in the world
- loss of trust in others, a sense that life is out of balance
- increased alcohol and drug use
- social withdrawal
- excitability, restlessness and nervousness
- pain complaints
- flulike and coldlike symptoms
- minimization of the traumatic incident
- hypervigilance
- feelings of shame, despair, hopelessness
- feelings of invulnerability, "spoiling for trouble"
- dizziness, trembling, light headedness
- rapid heartbeat
- feelings of euphoria

I asked them to go over the symptoms and see if any applied to their experience in the previous 2 weeks. Their reaction was impressive. Yes, of course, that was what they had been experiencing. Most were impressed with the similarities between the list and their own feelings at that time. During the next few days, I distributed the symptom list to several other community groups. The pattern of responses that I got was consistent.

Recognition for Larger Contact With the Community

At this point, it became apparent to me that the community, or, at least, a large part of the community, might possibly need psychological intervention. Since the symptoms were similar to those of trauma, and because much of the intervention work in trauma is educational, good public education via the media might be very effective. My goals would be the following:

1. validation of reality
2. education: predictability and normalization of response; empowerment
3. creation of a larger support system within Montreal

I then contacted a friend who is an editor of the English language newspaper (the *Montreal Gazette*) and explained the process of trauma response to her. I pointed out to her that in the last few weeks, I had become aware of how similar many people's reactions to the referendum were to symptoms of psychological trauma. I explained to her that a traumatic event is always regarded as a uniquely disruptive event in the life of affected individuals, families, and communities and that it required an appropriate response.

In a typical trauma situation, a community comes together to help comfort its victims. What had been happening in Quebec, however—at least as I heard it from the people whose data I had collected—was that many people were afraid to discuss their reactions because they were uncertain about the political position of their coworkers, friends, and other peers. This increased their sense of isolation. Another thing that happens in a typical trauma situation is that trained workers go into the setting and help the participants talk about their reactions through a variety of "debriefing" procedures. Obviously, this could not be done easily with an entire population, which is where I felt the media could help. By acknowledging the potential traumatic impact of the Referendum and by circulating the list of expected responses, we could help educate the public in the normalcy of their reactions at that time. We anticipated that this would reduce the isolation and fears of the extremely anxious part of the community. People needed also to understand that if they did experience these symptoms, they probably would not be of long duration.

We are all aware that education about the impact of trauma, normalization of the individual's response, and access to an appropriate support system are all important elements of trauma response. Without these functions, survivors may feel that their reaction is abnormal, and what might be contained as temporary distress can escalate to more permanent damage. The connection that takes place between people as result of trauma—natural disaster, community loss, and so on—can create a special intimacy that is the source of healing and a restoration of trust. This had not been possible here because of the continued sense of distrust and isolation.

The *Gazette's* response was to send a reporter to my class the following night to interview my students. The reporter then published the story about my students' reactions and those of others who we had interviewed. He added a little addendum. In his story he added the list of symptoms that I had been using, labeling them The Questions," and adding "Try Them." Besides that, he suggested to anyone who was interested that they fax their results to me.

Unfortunately, I had to leave Montreal to give an invited address in a different part of the world the day after the discussion with the press. I called my home as a matter of course and was told that it was impossible to enter the room where my fax machine was kept—it had been spewing out replies and comments from *Gazette* readers nonstop from early morning and throughout the day. It apparently touched a meaningful need in readers—the need for shared connection with others and the need for what became, even at a very simple level, a kind of mass debriefing.

Results

There were over 230 total responses, and I suspect, that if I had been home and able to replace the empty roll of fax printer paper, many more would have been included. The first goal-validation of the reality was about to be achieved. I was overwhelmed with the response. The quantitative response demonstrated that indeed people were showing many of the symptoms associated with posttraumatic stress. The *Montreal Gazette* published a story about the results on page one, upper right-hand column. The *Gazette* obviously thought they were significant, as well. In addition, the qualitative responses were of great value. They indicated that people were able to use the media as a mode of crisis intervention that allowed them to normalize and validate their experience. Here is some qualitative material from the questionnaire responses.

A 44-year-old woman wrote:

I was so relieved to read in today's *Gazette* that other people are and were as stressed by the referendum and its implications as I was. My husband and I were sitting there October 30, watching the results and feeling like a couple of too tightly strung piano strings ready to give at any moment, and although relieved to have the 'no' side win, it was not a feeling of happiness but rather sadness that the entire country had been put through such torture—and for what?

A 50-year-old male wrote:

Finally there is an article that addresses the issues of psychological wounds relating to the referendum process. . . . This questionnaire, I'm happy to say, is a kind of therapy for me, for it allows an opportunity to express feelings that have been bottled up inside that were to some extent still felt as a result of the referendum. It gave us silent voices a way of expressing feelings that have (previously) only been expressed within the confines of the family.

And another:

Thank you for your article. It was quite enlightening. I thought I was going crazy. I have the added stress of working in a bank. The more people came in and transferred money out of our province, the more heated the discussions or shall I say comments about the panicking idiots who don't know what they're doing. It was quite unbearable, and I was drawn to tears many times. Even our customers noticed the atmosphere. I hope the politicians realize what they are doing to the people of the province.

A woman wrote:

I am a French speaking Quebecois, and I was treated as a dog by my coworkers because I was not for the 'yes.' They made me feel that I did not belong in the French-speaking society. They ejected me because I did not agree with them. I was really afraid and worried. My whole world was falling apart, and I could not do anything about it.

We know that empowerment is another goal of trauma response. This was reflected in the comments of a 51-year-old woman who wrote: "Hope this is of some help. If there is any group, organization or movement, or force that can counteract the present unhappy state, count me in."

Lack of naturally occurring support was reflected in many stories about neighbors not talking to each other. One woman from a small town outside of Montreal told of a baby-sitter who had been sitting for her children for many years. After the referendum, the woman refused to talk to her or to baby-sit again, because they had been on opposite sides of the vote. One man said: "The thing I currently notice is that despite the referendum being over, there is an obvious feeling of relief on the 'No' side but an over-all feeling of alienation from one another. . . . We work together, play to-gether, yet we are totally apart in our differences and silent about them."

As soon as this story was published, it was picked up by radio and tel-evision reporters all over Quebec and Canada and far beyond those borders. My subsequent work with radio and television programs was to respond to these findings and to meet the second and third goals of the media use, as described earlier.

Another part of the situation which was reported was a sense of isola-tion from the rest of the world. People reported that Americans and others in the world could not understand what all of the fuss was about, and they denied the quality of their painful experience. As the international press soon became involved (we were interviewed by *Psychology Today, Harper's Magazine,* the *Washington Post,* the *Boston Globe, The International Herald Tribune,* and the *Manchester Guardian,* amongst others,) this situation di-minished, and the sense of isolation from the rest of the world decreased. As Kate Johnson of *Psychology Today* described the situation, "Canadian seismologists described nothing unusual last October. But psychologists in Quebec monitored tremors of earthquake proportions. And the aftershocks continue" (March/April, 1996).

Another positive outcome was an interview I did for the *Canadian Journal of Family Practice,* which goes to all family practitioners in Canada. This helped the practitioners to respond to patients who were experiencing what was being called "Referendum stress" or "Anglo angst."

This experience can teach us at least three important things. These in-clude the following:

- the use of the media in general
- the double impact of trauma work and the media
- the importance of interactive communication through the media

As professionals, we can learn yet again of the value of the media in bringing our message to the public. It is of value when we can tune into the public's reactions, feelings, and needs and then respond appropriately. Psychologists and other professionals who work in the field of trauma have ready access to the media and should take advantage of the value of that ac-cess. Of particular interest to me in this situation was the power of interac-tive use of the media. While nothing can ever fully replace the impact of a person-to-person interaction, having the public interact with us through the use of the media can still be very powerful. With increasing use of the Internet, this is of greater impact in our work.

This experience clearly demonstrated that, in this kind of political unrest, with all of its associated turmoil, the appropriate use of the media by psychologists and other mental-health workers can provide a beneficial educational function to the public.

THE CLERGY CONNECTION

Responding to traumas, particularly community-based situations, is frequently based on a short-term intervention/prevention model. This model consists most frequently of an immediate outpouring of aid, both material and psychological. Often, this assistance drops off after the immediate situation has passed. The community can then be left to complete its healing using only its inherent resource people, who sometimes do not have much formal training in trauma response. In addition, because of their own involvement in the first stage, these well-intentioned individuals may now be suffering from their own secondary or vicarious traumatization. The goal of this project was to intervene after the immediate response had passed and short-term helpers had gone. At that time, we felt the need to identify that part of the helper population that could follow up with the community (with appropriate training).

We explored several communities of different sizes and decided that perhaps one of the most overlooked resources was the clergy.

Having identified this group, we needed to test a medium that would allow both psychologists and intrinsic caregivers in any part of North America to interact with each other.

Initial research identified the clergy as a group not only in need of our services, but also open to working with us. The mechanics of the second issue were worked out by developing a familiarity and comfort level with "bridge lines," a form of teleconferencing that allows several people to interact simultaneously on existing telephone lines. This proved to be a new, valuable, and relatively underdeveloped aspect of the psychologists' role. Each week, we would meet with clergy from different part of North America via bridge line and help them to identify their roles in traumatic situations. Each had different experiences to contribute, and all of them reported that they felt a sense of isolation and a need to connect with others in their fields.

Finally, at the end of the project, we connected all of the participants together on our bridge line and helped them to link up with each other. They were all very grateful for the experiences, and they reinforced our feeling that this is not only a relatively untouched group of helpers, but also a group that needs to stay in close touch with each other to share their burdens.

ANIMALS AND HEALING

Throughout this book, we have been emphasizing the need to help build on our clients' strengths. We have demonstrated how an individual can become a "Phoenix" with the right combination of appropriate qualities of support at crucial times. There are, however, other, perhaps less traditional, sources of support that can be of great help to us and to our clients as we struggle through this new, difficult period in our history.

One of the external sources of support that some of us may overlook can be the gifts we can receive from animals. Not all of us will be able to respond positively to this statement. Some may have had frightening experiences as children and held on to the fears that were generated then; others may have allergies. Nevertheless, we feel that some of the experiences we will demonstrate below may be of help.

At the one year anniversary of September 11, 2001 (9-11), Larry M. Hawke, DVM (Dr. of Veterinary Medicine), President and CEO of the American Society for the Prevention of Cruelty to Animals (ASPCA) started his newsletter with this statement: "Great occasions do not make heroes or cowards; they simply unveil us. Silently and imperceptibly, as we wake or sleep, we grow strong or weak; and at last some crisis shows what we have become." He goes on to acknowledge the bravery of the ASPCA's humane law enforcement officers and medical personnel. He tells his story:

> I watched the first evening (September 11, 2001) as our officers escorted the first of several groups of worried pet parents to their apartments around ground zero. I'll never forget one of the first people whose pets we helped rescue. Our officers had to go up 10 flights of stairs in the dark with only flashlights to guide them. There was no electricity in any of the buildings and therefore no elevators!
>
> Later that evening a man named Frank came back with one of our officers, smiling ear to ear. He jumped out of the car holding his two cats, showering them with hugs and kisses. What he said next will stay with me for a lifetime. He said "Thank you very much for helping me rescue my four-legged family members! They mean so very much to me, especially since my wife is still missing!"

The New York City Port Authority Police were escorting groups of grief-stricken families by boat from Pier 94 directly to Ground Zero. Each trip on the boat had two or three pet-assisted therapy dog teams to comfort grieving family members. Since I had lost my sister, I personally experienced the memorial boat ride to Ground Zero.

I watched the families with tearful eyes, clutching flowers, teddy bears and photographs of their loved ones as they boarded the boat. Chaplains from the Red Cross and other counseling staff accompanied us on the ride along with tail-wagging therapists. I watched family members break down with grief as they viewed the still-burning towers, leaving behind their pictures and flowers. They could hardly see though the tears but I always saw their tears turn to smiles, at least for a moment, when one of the therapy dogs nuzzled up alongside of them. They could not help but be spiritually lifted when they began hugging the dogs with their tails wagging. These dogs and their human handlers were silent heroes of this disaster, working behind the scenes, helping those that needed it most during very emotional times (from a letter from Larry M. Hawke; used with his permission).

At the anniversary memorial service held at Ground Zero 1 year after 9-11, a rescue dog was present and felt to be of great help. A New York City firehouse has also created a canine memorial.

One of my own more touching experiences was with my dog Mello, a 1-year-old abused Labrador that we retrieved from the SPCA pound. She was permitted to stay in my office during sessions, provided that the client invited her in. Once there, she had to lie down next to my chair, across the room from the client, and go to sleep. She was deeply asleep in that position one day when an extremely traumatized young woman was having her session. Quite suddenly, the woman, who was sitting at a considerable distance from Mello, started to weep silently. Mello immediately awoke from her sleep, gently went over to the client, licked (Mello's version of kissing) the client's legs and arms. She had simply administered her own personal prescription for healing. There are no human words that can replace that intensely moving moment, nor are there any better ways of expressing what this innocent canine/therapist expressed so poignantly and spontaneously.

One of my dog-run colleagues told me that on 9-11, as she lay on her bed watching the disaster unfold, she wept silently. Her dog joined her and licked her face, most sympathetically. Again, this is an instance of administering canine healing.

A study by Allen, Blascovich, and Mendes (2002) found that the presence of a pet mitigates the effect of stressors on heart rate and blood pressure and hastens recovery to baselines. Pets were found to lower stress by providing nonjudgmental companionship.

Dr. Alan Beck, Director of the Center for the Human-Animal Bond at Purdue University and coauthor of *Between Pets and People: The Importance of Animal Companionship,* tells us that "when you interact with animals you typically have a relaxation response. There's a drop in blood pressure and you feel calmer. It's a pure tactile focus of attention when you pet them, and that's more relaxing than doing 'nothing' with your thoughts."

My own experiences have enlarged my understanding of the importance of pets in a variety of settings. One Sunday morning, I took my Mello for her walk through the park quite early, around 7:30 AM, a time when very few people are about. As we came out of the park, she ran a bit ahead of me, and as we turned a corner, I realized that she had greeted an old woman who was walking alone. The woman, who was considerably older than myself, was not very well dressed. I told her that I hoped that Mello had not bothered her. She said "No, not at all," and then, quite spontaneously, she said "Meeting your dog was a pleasure. I love dogs, and meeting Mello made me feel much less all alone in the world."

When we think of the importance of support systems in our work in healing, think, if you will, of the impact of a simple, loving pet in the life of a lonely person, particularly a person who may be frightened or traumatized by a suddenly changing world.

Remember, also, that the numbers of older people in our world is increasing dramatically, and many of these seniors are very lonely. As the level of ongoing trauma and terrorism increases in a world with lonely adults, the combination of new, frightening experiences and diminishing support systems can impede their ability to respond in a resilient manner. As the world simultaneously creates both new fears and new needs to depend upon the "kindness of strangers," companion animals may become one of our more valuable assets. Learning how to interact with, teach, and work with these animals can easily become a valuable part of the training of any potential crisis or trauma worker.

REFERENCES

Allen, K. A., Blascovich, J., & Mendes, W. B. (2002). *Psychosomatic Medicine, 64*(5). Quoted in APA's *Monitor on Psychology, 33*(11).

Beck, A., & Katcher, A. (1996). *Between pets and people: The importance of animal companionship.* West Lafayette, IN: Purdue University Press.

Johnson, K. (1996, March/April). "Separation anxiety." *Psychology Today.*

Menninger, K. *The man.* In memory of Dr. Karl A. Menninger July 22, 1893–July 18, 1990 by Stannle Anderson Topeka Capital Journal 7/19/1990.

Wainrib, B., & Bloch, E. (1998). *Crisis intervention and trauma response: Theory and practice.* New York: Springer Publishing.

Wainrib, B., & Haber, S. (2000). *Men, women and prostate cancer: A medical and psychological guide for women and the men they love.* Oakland, CA: New Harbinger Publications.

CHAPTER 11

Forgiveness

It is easy to love those who love us. It is difficult to like those who are critical of us. Yet it is crucial to forgive those who hurt us. Forgiveness is a challenge, but countless people are able to meet the challenge. . . . They say "You have controlled me in the past. But now, you can't control me any more. I decide how I want to live."

—V. P. Sharma (Mind, 1996)

If we really want to love, we must learn how to forgive.

—Mother Theresa

Having written so much about our inhumanity to each other throughout this book, I now come to grips with a concept about which I admit my ambivalence: forgiveness for perpetrators of traumas. However, it is obvious that if the kinds of traumas that we have reviewed in this book continue to be created throughout the world without some kind of healing mechanism, we will eventually regress to the level of cave dwellers.

In a previous chapter however, I found myself writing:

What we needed at that moment (9-11) was a sense of a safe place, either within ourselves or in the outside world, and a good support network of people who were able to empathize, talk, listen, and understand. More than anything else, we needed forgiveness. We needed forgiveness of our own frailties, forgiveness of the fact that we had been blessed with being survivors and alive.

Even the most horrendous of crimes cannot be allowed to sustain permanent hatred. The recent visit of the Chancellor of Germany to the State of Israel and, most particularly, his visit to the memorial for the six million

Jews killed by the Nazis, is a moving example that, for life to go on, at some level, there has to be some kind of forgiving. Nobel Peace Laureate Elie Wiesel sang Germany's praises for observing remembrance for Holocaust victims. But he urged the German parliament to go farther to seek forgiveness for the Third Reich's behavior. "We desperately want to have hope for the new century," he declared. Recently, German President Johannes Rau asked the Israeli Knesset (i.e., Congress) for forgiveness for the Holocaust (Wright, 2005).

The existence of the Truth and Reconciliation Commission in South Africa attests to changes in the thinking about forgiveness as well. And the broad undertaking of the Gacaca process by Pearlman, Staub and others in Rwanda as described in an earlier chapter, is another important step in the same direction.

MOVEMENTS TOWARD FORGIVENESS

The establishment of the Truth and Reconciliation Commission in South Africa was the first move on a national scale for a nation to reconcile with its internal oppressors. Archbishop Desmond Tutu is the Chairman of the commission. Earlier in this book, I described the moving experience I had when the commission was inaugurated in Capetown. Archbishop Tutu has written (2003) that

> forgiveness is not being sentimental. The study of forgiveness has become a growth industry. Whereas previously it was something often dismissed pejoratively as spiritual and religious, now, because of developments such as the Truth and Reconciliation Commission in South Africa, it is gaining attention as an academic discipline studied by psychologists, and theologians. . . . Forgiving means abandoning your right to pay back your perpetrator in his own coin, but it is a loss that liberates the victim. In the Truth and Reconciliation Commission we heard people speak of a sense of relief after forgiving.

When the wrongdoer does confess and the victim does forgive, it does not mean that it is the end of the process. Most frequently the wrong has affected the victim in tangible, material ways. Apartheid provided the Whites with enormous benefits and privileges, leaving its victims deprived and exploited. If someone steals my pen and then asks me to forgive him, unless he returns my pen the sincerity of his contrition and confession will be considered to be nil. Confession, forgiveness and reparation, wherever feasible, form a part of a continuum (*IONS Review,* 2003).

Because of my own admitted ambivalence, let us refer to several people who have very strong convictions in this area.

Dr. Marc Schulz, a psychologist at Bryn Mawr College, has researched forgiveness and has found that "Each time we witness an act of forgiveness, we marvel at its power to heal, to break a seemingly unending cycle of pain." Forgiveness is something virtually all people aspire to: 94% surveyed in a nationwide Gallup poll said it was important to forgive; however, it is not something we frequently offer. In the same survey, only 48% said they usually tried to forgive others (2004). Perhaps this is because forgiveness is something we don't fully understand.

PHYSIOLOGICAL COMPONENTS
OF FORGIVENESS

In an effort to understand the physiological as well as the psychological components of forgiveness, I recently contacted Dr. T. F. Farrow in Sheffield, England. He has contributed interesting research about forgiveness which has a special perspective. He was very helpful and forthcoming about his work in this field. He says "The survival of Homo Sapiens depends upon the avoidance of unnecessary conflict though mechanisms such as forgiveness" (in Farrow, YingZhang, & Wilkinson, 2001). He describes forgiveness as comprising "multiple cognitive components. One such component may be to judge the forgivability of another's actions. Another component may be the ability to empathize with others, including an aggressor" (p. 2436). Farrow describes empathy as consisting of two components: "An affective (visceral emotional reaction) and a cognitive (understanding of the conspecific's behavior). Empathy and forgiveness are both heavily dependent on the expression and interpretation of emotions" (p. 2436).

Defining forgiveness as "Ceasing to feel angry or resentful towards another," Dr. Farrow used MRI scans "To examine neural correlates of making empathic and forgivability judgements," and adds, "To our knowledge this is the first study to examine the functional anatomy of forgiveness. We posited that forgiveness incorporates judgments of another's intentions, their emotional states and the forgivability of their actions" (p. 2436). He used the MRIs to detect brain regions engaged by judging others' emotional states and forgivability of their crimes. In one study, he instructed 10 volunteers to read and make judgments "based on social scenarios and a high level baseline task" (i.e., social reasoning).

Both empathic and forgivability judgements activated areas of the brain that were different from those activated by empathic judgements. Empathic judgements also activated left anterior middle temporal and left inferior frontal gyri, while forgivability judgements activated posterior singulate gyros. Empathic and forgivability judgements activate specific regions of the human brain, which we propose contribute to social cohesion (p. 2437).

Dr. Farrow's (2001) research enforces the information that there is "an emerging literature on the beneficial effects of forgiveness as a psychotherapeutic intervention for many conditions (e.g., posttraumatic stress disorder)." His research results gave "a strong indication that activations of very high level cognitive process are recordable, and that mental status could be reasonably predicted to show differing patterns of activation which may be amenable to normalization through cognitive intervention" (p. 2438).

Nancy A. Peddle is a psychologist who did her research on forgiveness. She (2001) writes, "At the core of both trauma recovery and forgiveness is a perceived traumatic event or betrayal. Both recovery and forgiveness are linked to the end of human suffering, alleviation of anxiety, depression and hopelessness." She describes the act of telling one's story "with all the emotions and heartache" as a way to help the victim of violence shift to being a survivor. She interviewed 90 adolescent and adult war refugees who ranged in age from 13 to 85. They had experienced wars in the Balkans, Africa, or World War II. "Their stories contained the horrors usually found only in nightmares, full of the atrocities of "ethnic cleansing," rape, torture, brutal beatings, mass killings in the ovens of Auschwitz, and witnessing the cold blooded killing of relatives and friends." Her interviews with these people revealed that "betrayal was at the root of the trauma and, for some, forgiveness transformed and healed them." Her results showed a relationship between forgiveness and recovery/resilience. "Those who were forgiving and those who said they were forgiving were more recovered and resilient, as demonstrated by their hope and their reconnecting with their selves and their communities."

She also tells us that "the ability to forgive is a function of maturation and experience. . . . Optimally, forgiveness would become one factor in part of trauma recovery (and) should be a part of a common strategy for social change in the aftermath of such gross injustices."

Perhaps, as Friedrich Nietzsche said, we associate forgiveness with weakness. Or perhaps we view forgiveness as an almost saintly quality that imbues only the very special and assume that it most certainly cannot be learned. Those of us who work in the helping professions know that forgiveness can be learned. And those of us who have survived long-term marriages certainly know that forgiveness is an essential piece of the formula for sustaining them! In order for a marriage to endure, we have to learn not only how to repent but how to react to others repentance. This model goes far beyond that of marriages, but as so many things, learning begins at home. Perhaps the art of forgiveness is as much in learning how to recognize it in others, as it is about learning how to create it. In interpersonal relationships, the art of repentance is unique to each of us. It may frequently be nonverbal; it may sometimes be active, but just as often, it may be passive.

Robert Grant (1999) reminds us that

> victims of trauma are by definition "overwhelmed and rendered help-
> less." They are unable to weather the shock and impact of their injuries.
> They need support and guidance. Trauma exposes aspects of external and
> internal reality that have been previously unacknowledged. . . . Old an-
> swers no longer suffice. Priorities are reordered. Concerns about identity,
> the value of suffering, the importance of justice and the appropriateness
> of forgiveness are figural. Recognizing the amount of evil and cruelty in
> the world, along with the impact these realities have for images of God
> and the value of human relationship, demand careful consideration and
> continual reflection. Questions of identity proliferate. Responses to these
> demands require more comprehensive ways of taking up life. Without
> support, guidance and reflection, it is almost impossible to develop new
> frames of meaning capable of incorporating the life truths exposed by the
> experience of trauma (p. E2).

An organization called the International Forgiveness Institute has de-
veloped a program about forgiveness for children in Belfast, Ireland. We are all aware of the long-term painful conflict that residents of this area have experienced. The University of Wisconsin is researching the Ireland program for the development of forgiveness education in the schools of Belfast. Working with young children would appear to be one of the most hopeful means of preventing the repetition of the bloodied political horrors that that country has undergone. The children are being taught bet-
ter ways to handle their conflicts, based on the principles of forgiveness. The International Forgiveness Institute, which reports on this project, has a Web site (hhht://www.forgivenessday.org/steps–to-forgiveness.html), which is very helpful.

Fred Luskin is the director and founder of the Stanford University Forgiveness Project, a group that conducts forgiveness training and research. He says:

I define forgiveness as the experience of peace and understanding that can be felt at the present moment. You forgive by challenging the rigid rules you have for other people's behavior and by focusing on the good things in your life as opposed to the bad. Forgiveness does not mean forgetting or denying that painful things occurred. Forgiveness is the powerful assertion that bad things will not ruin your today even though they may have spoiled your past (1996, p. 12).

Luskin teaches us that:

The process of forgiveness can be a liberating experience; one that if practiced proactively, can lead to a wonderful experience of life. Interestingly, forgiveness can only occur because we have been given the gift of the ability to make choices. We have the choice to forgive or not to forgive and no one can force us to do either. Conversely, if we want to forgive someone, no one can stop us no matter how poorly they may act. This ability to forgive is a manifestation of the personal control we have over our lives. It is nice to reflect upon and feel the respect that e have been given to be able to make such profound choices (1996, p. 13).

While this approach may not be comfortable for all of our readers, Luskin adds:

Compellingly, the option to forgive also implies that we had discretion as to whether or not we took offense in the first place. While forgiving may be a difficult enough choice for many of us, imagine how our lives would be if we rarely or never used our power of choice to take offense. Since we have choice, wouldn't it make sense to limit the amount of times we are hurt or offended so that the need to forgive rarely if ever arises? The ability to live life without taking offense, without giving blame, and by offering forgiveness are choices that offer a life of great peace (1996, p. 13).

Luskin has identified several scientific studies that reveal the following:

- People who are more forgiving report fewer health problems.
- Forgiveness leads to less stress.
- Failure to forgive may be more important than hostility as a risk factor for heart disease.
- People who blame other people for their troubles have higher incidence of illness such as cardiovascular disease and cancer.
- People who imagine not forgiving someone show negative changes in blood pressure, muscle tension and immune response.
- People who imagine forgiving their offender note immediate improvement in their cardiovascular, muscular and nervous systems.

POPULARITY OF THE CONCEPT OF FORGIVENESS

So popular has the concept of forgiveness become that the worldwide Web presents us with such products as the "Forgiveness Web," which offers "The Apology Room," a message board, and "Forgiveness and the Media." An organization called the Worldwide Forgiveness Alliance is seeking to establish the first global holiday, International Forgiveness Day, to be celebrated on the first Sunday of every August, beginning in 2005.

The Alliance has published a list of 17 steps to forgiveness. Included are such items as the following:

- confront your emotional pain, fear anger and grief.
- realize that the forgiveness can only be appropriate after you have processed your fear, anger and grief.
- start releasing anger, sadness, grief and fear (using) any processes, therapies, and therapists available.

Dr. Robert Coles tells us, in an Internet piece, that he thinks "forgiveness is an aspect of our humanity. I think a lot of us are brought up to believe that if we don't somehow forgive, whatever it is that's ailing, troubling, angering, enraging or shaming us, or getting us in any way worked up, is going to live longer without our forgiveness whether it's ourselves or others we are forgiving" (Forgiveness.org).

WHEN FORGIVENESS BACKFIRES

A paper by Kristi Gordon, PhD, called "The Risk of Forgiveness: Predicting Women in Domestic Violence Shelters' Intentions to Return to Their Partners," contains material that we should take into consideration.

Gordon tells us that "whereas it is likely that social and economic constraints play a role in a woman's decision to return to an abusive relationship, it is also apparent that psychological and emotional factors may influence this decision as well."

As many of us have observed in our practices, some of these women value the experience of being in a relationship over their own personal safety. Hence, "forgiveness" per se can have both negative and positive effects. Unfortunately, we have very little research on this very sensitive topic.

Gordon further comments on this subject, "If a woman is able to forgive her partner's behavior, then she might be more likely to desire to return to the relationship."

A recent finding on dating violence indicates that "young women who blame themselves for violent episodes are more likely to state that they would forgive violent episodes from their male partners and indicate a higher likelihood of staying in an abusive relationship" (Katz, Street, & Arias, 1997, p. 265).

A recent article in the *Psychotherapy Networker* (2004, p. 23) reports a study by psychologist Jennie Noll of the University of Cincinnati. Noll has found that if forgiveness involves reconciling with the abuser, it may cause more psychological problems. She compared 55 sexually abused women with 65 women who suffered other significant childhood trauma, such as physical assault or . . . family conflict. She found that:

> sexually abused women who had progressed through internal forgiveness—letting go of their anger and desire for revenge and moving on with their lives—showed significant reduction in anxiety, PTSD symptoms and dissociation. But those women who were focused externally and were trying to reconcile with their abusive fathers fared worse in the reduction of their anxiety [and] women who had suffered childhood trauma other than sexual abuse showed no ill-effects from attempting to reconcile.

She adds, "In general forgiveness does seem to be an adaptive process. Savvy therapists shouldn't avoid the work of forgiveness, but they shouldn't automatically equate forgiveness with reconciliation" (p. 23).

Dr. Everett Worthington, Chair of the Department of Psychology of Virginia Commonwealth University, is the executive director of A Campaign for Forgiveness Research. Dr. Worthington (2003) writes, "Resentment, one of the core elements of unforgiveness, is like carrying around a red-hot rock with the intention of someday throwing it back at the one that hurt you. It tires us and burns us. Who wouldn't want simply to let the rock fall to the ground?" (p. 9).

In a presentation I made several years ago to celebrate a notable anniversary, I said:

> We create our own darkness, in our failures at connection with each other, even in the best intentioned relationship. However, when we have experienced times of joy and contact, we learn that with the right ingredients, such as support and understanding, we can use the darkness as a turning point, a jumping-off point for further growth" (Wainrib, 2001).

In the final analysis, I will leave you with the words of Luskin (1996) and those of Buddha: "Even people with devastating losses can learn to forgive and feel better psychologically and emotionally" (Luskin, p. 12). And Buddha's eternal wisdom shines through in the following: "You will not be punished for your anger. You will be punished by your anger."

REFERENCES

Coles, R. "A Campaign for Forgiveness Research." Forgiving.org

Farrow, T. F. D., YingZhang, I. D, & Wilkinson, I. D., Spence. S. A., Deakin. J. F. W., Tarrier, N., & Griffiths, P. D. (2001, August). Investigating the functional anatomy of empathy and forgiveness. *Neuroreport, 12.*

Gordon, K. "The risk of forgiveness: Predicting women in domestic violence shelters intentions to return to their partners." Retrieved October, 2003, from Forgiving.org

Grant, R. (1999). Spirituality and trauma: An essay. *Traumatology, 5*(1), E2.

Katz, J., Street, A. E., & Arias, I. (1997). Individual differences in self-appraisals and responses to dating violence. *Violence and Victims, 12,* 265– 276.

Luskin, F. (1996, Sept./Oct.). Four steps of forgiveness. *Healing Currents Magazine.*

Mother Theresa: Mother Theresa's message to fourth UN Woman's Conference.

Nietzsche, F. (1917). *Beyond good and evil.* New York: Boni and Liveright Publishers.

Noll, J., in G. Cooper. (2004).The happiness wars. *Psychotherapy Networker, 28*(6), 23.

Peddle, N. A. (2001, December). "Forgiveness in recovery/resiliency from the trauma of war among a selected group of adolescents and adult refugees." Dissertation Abstracts International: Section B: The Sciences & Engineering, Vol. 62(5-B), 225.

Schulz, M. S., Cowan, P. A., Cowan, C. P., & Brennan, R. T. (2004). Coming home upset: Gender, marital satisfaction, and the daily spillover of workday experience into couple interactions. *Journal of Family Psychology, 18,* 250–263.

Schulz, M. S., Cowan, P. A., et al. (2004). Coming home upset: Gender, marital satisfaction, and the daily spillover of workday experience into couple interactions. *Journal of Family Psychology, 18*(1), 250– 263.

Sharma, V. P. (1996). *Mind.* California: Hay House.

Tutu, D. (2003, September/November). *IONS Review,* p. 15.

Wainrib B. (2001). Special presentation, Post 9-11 Montreal, Quebec.

Worldwide Forgiveness Alliance, p. 9. Retrieved April 2, 2005, from http://www.forgivenessday.org/steps-to-forgiveness.html

Worthington, E. (2003). *National Science Review, 11.*

Wright, R. (2005). Telling the Truth Project.

CHAPTER 12

Final Thoughts

Throughout this journey of exploration of varieties of traumatic experiences and approaches to healing, we have been quoting some very wise folks. As we attempt to recover the pain and healing of body mind and spirit, it is appropriate that we end with yet more meaningful words of wisdom.

Here is an age-old Sufi story:

Some [people] bought an elephant, which they exhibited in a dark shed. As seeing it with the eye was impossible, every one felt it with the palm of his hand. The hand of one fell on the trunk: He said "this animal is like a water-pipe." Another touched its ear. To him the creature seemed like a fan. Another handled its leg and described the elephant as having the shape of a pillar. Another stroked its back. "Truly," he said, "this elephant resembles a throne."

Had each of them held a lighted candle, there would have been no contradiction in their words. The essence of our work is to light candles for those in the darkness of trauma. At the same time, we must always remember to nourish our own souls

Long ago, Rabbi Kook (1865–1935), chief rabbi of the settlement in Palestine, wrote:

So long as the world moves along accustomed paths, so long as there are no wild catastrophes, we can find sufficient substance for our lives by contemplating surface events, theories and movements of society. We can acquire inner richness from this external kind of "property." But this is not the case when life encounters fiery forces of evil and chaos. Then the "revealed" world begins to totter. Then we who try to sustain ourselves

only from the surface aspects of existence will suffer terrible impoverish-
ment, begin to stagger. . . . Then we will feel welling up within ourselves
a burning thirst for that inner substance and vision that transcends the
obvious surfaces of existence and remains unaffected by the world's
catastrophes. From such inner sources we will seek the waters of joy,
which can quicken the dry outer skeleton of existence (Sermon, 1932).

No one says this better than the German poet, Rainer Maria Rilke:

Do not think that he who seeks to comfort you lives untroubled among
the simple quiet words that sometimes do you good. His [sic] life has
much difficulty and sorrow. Were it otherwise he would never have been
able to find those words.

And we close with the words of wisdom, once again, of David Elkins:
"The authentic therapist is a lit candle of being that lights the candle that
has gone out in the client's soul" (1998, p. 185).

REFERENCES

Elkins, D. (1998). *Beyond religion*. Illinois: Quest Books.
Kook, Rabbi, Chief Rabbi of settlement in Palestine. (1865–1935).
Rilke, R. M. (1903). *Letters to a young poet*. New York: Modern Library.

Index